It's Not About The Food

A Woman's Guide To Making Peace With Food and Our Bodies

Esther Kane, MSW

www.estherkane.com
www.endyoureatingdisorder.com

Library and Archives Canada Cataloguing in Publication

Kane, Esther, 1971-

It's not about the food: a woman's guide to making peace with food and our bodies / by Esther Kane.

Includes bibliographical references.

ISBN 978-0-9780706-2-5

1. Eating disorders in women. 2. Women--Psychology. 3. Kane, Esther, 1971-. I. Title.

RC552.E18K36 2009   616.85'260082   C2008-907654-0

ISBN 978-0-9780706-2-5

If you would like to publish sections of this book, please contact the publisher for permission.

Published by:
Esther Kane, MSW
250.338.1800
www.estherkane.com
esther@estherkane.com

Cover design by E-magination Design: www.emagnination.ca

Cover illustration
& content design by Bobbie Cann: www.canndesign.com

Cover typeface "Enchanted Prairie Dog" designed by
Shoshanna : users.cwnet.com/shoshana/serendipity.html

other books by esther kane

Dump That Chump: A Ten-Step Plan to Ending Bad Relationships and Attracting the Fabulous Partner You Deserve
Available at: www.dumpthatchump.com

What Your Mama Can't or Won't Teach You: Grown Women's Stories of Their Teen Years
Available at: www.guidebooktowomanhood.com

dedication

To all of the amazing women I have met along my own journey to finding peace with food and my body – you are all gifts to me and I cherish each and every one of you. When I help you, you help me and that is the beauty of the work I have been given the privilege of doing in this life. My hope is that we all continue to find the peace, self-love and joy that are our birthright and that we pass this on to future generations of women so that they don't have to struggle as we have.

contents

introduction

I want to start this book by telling you my own personal story.

Why, you ask? Well, there are a number of reasons one of which is that I, too, have been through my own personal hell when it comes to food and body image. It is my hope that, knowing my story will help you, my reader, to benefit from the advice offered in the pages that follow because their author *knows whereof she speaks.*

Secondly, as a psychotherapist, I know intimately that sharing one's story can be both cathartic and healing. Every day, in my office, I hear other women's stories – stories of struggle and suffering that end in triumph – and, every day, I am inspired by these stories and filled with admiration for these women who, through inner strength, turn their struggle into self-understanding and, yes, even wisdom.

Perhaps by sharing my own story, I too can offer hope and inspiration to women in the midst of their struggle with food and body image. This is a novel concept for me. I'm usually the one sitting in the opposite chair, quietly nodding my head, showing empathy and concern, listening intently while revealing very little about myself.

I want to preface my story and everything I'm about to say by acknowledging that not everything you are about to read is flattering, either to me or my family. A lot of personal work and a long, intense involvement in my own therapy process have brought me to where I am today. In the process, a great deal has been healed. I have been healed of the past and have been able to let go of the things that kept me from being myself.

Today, I can honestly say, I am fully aware that my parents did the best they could with what they were given and that they love me very much and always have. As an adult, I have become acutely aware of their struggles and their own childhood situations and both understand and appreciate how these may have led them to choose the parenting style they did in raising me. As a result of my own struggles, I have only compassion for what they have endured and survived.

About myself, I have learned that I've been scared my whole life – scared of everything and everyone around me – and that, frankly, I'm sick and tired of living this way. This is what I have discovered is at the very core of my "eating disorder" – fear. I've come to learn that fear is a killer of life and that, if not confronted head on, will cripple you until the day you really do die.

I don't want to be one of those people about whom it can be said: "She had so much potential." I don't want to live in fear. I want to be brave and courageous and sail uncharted seas. For me, those uncharted seas represent the depths of who I used to be, who I am now and who I want to become in the future – they are the uncharted seas of myself.

This, for me, is a scary adventure but an exciting one. I'm determined to become and continue being, for the remainder of the time that is given me, the person I want to be. And I won't let fear get in the way of doing what I need to do to set myself free. Telling my story, my truth, is a part – indeed, a critical part – of the adventure before me; and for you, if you choose to come along. It is my hope that hearing my story will inspire you to do the same and to set yourself free – free from obsessing about food and weight and what you look like, and then, layer-by-layer, free from everything that's hidden underneath, everything that lurks below the surface and prevents you from being all that you can be.

Let's get started, shall we?

Big hugs,

Esther

1
my story

I'm not going to tell you my WHOLE story (this is not an auto-biography, after all) but I do want to tell you, in chronological order, the history of my eating disorder. As I write this, I am a thirty-seven year old, professional woman who is mostly (I repeat, mostly) healed from an illness that nearly cost me my life. For this, I am extremely grateful and amazed. I make my living by helping other women heal from their dysfunctional relationships with food and body image and this work, my work, is more rewarding than words can possibly describe.

I am happily married to a man I adore, someone who is my best friend and partner in life. We have a lovely house, two fabulous Siberian kitty-cats, Abe and Ike, our substitute babies (they do the job nicely, thank you), and I own my office, which has plenty of light and high ceilings and overlooks a river. We live on a beautiful island off the west coast of Canada where life is slow-paced and peaceful. We have wonderful friends, many hobbies and good health. Not too shabby, I must confess. Life is pretty sweet, indeed. But it wasn't always this way.

I was born in May of 1971 in North Bay, Ontario. My parents were young hippies from London, England who had recently transplanted themselves in Canada. Like many children of my generation, my parents divorced when I was young, four and a half to be exact.

Hence, my first real loss in my short life had taken place and it was devastating. I grew up as an only child so I didn't have any siblings to lean on or fight with; it was just my mum and I.

I saw my dad on weekends He had moved into an apartment downtown in this "groovy" new high-rise that had a swimming pool in the basement. To a four-year-old, this was Nirvana! I remember lots of orange and brown, typically 70's, décor and that my dad had bought a special loveseat that pulled out into a cozy little bed perfect for a little person like me. Because my mother had done all of the cooking when they were together, we ate out a lot. At a very young age, I learned to use chopsticks at a Chinese-Canadian restaurant in my dad's neighbourhood – a great party trick as it turned out. To my delight, I was regularly served Chef Boyardee ravioli with meat sauce out of a can! It wasn't long before I discovered that I could get away with eating dessert at daddy's place, then go to mummy's house and get another dessert! I soon learned to lie about food – a trick I thought was brilliant at the time but later caused me a great deal of grief.

For the next three years, I lived with my mum during the week and my dad on the weekends. At this time, my mother discovered her incredible flair for writing about food and began writing for some high-end Toronto publications. My mother, by the way, is a gastronomical genius. She is pure brilliance in the kitchen, able to create delicious gourmet fare with the greatest of ease, and has impeccable tastes. No matter what the cuisine –

French, Chinese or Persian – mum can always discern between the exquisite and the not-so-exquisite. Thanks to this talent, she eventually became a star food editor/columnist and took me along on all of her restaurant reviews. She taught me the difference between cheap, oily French fries and crispy, thin, and elegant "frites". And who would have thought? This little girl loved being a "food snob" as much as she loved Chef Boyardee!

Around this same time, my father dated a woman who was a staunch vegetarian and this opened up a whole new world to him. He stopped eating meat and became zealous about preventing cruelty to animals and professed that being vegan (not eating any animal products, including dairy and honey products) was the best way to save the earth. He soon became Macrobiotic – what he later jokingly referred to as "Macroneurotic".

For those of you who don't already know, the Macrobiotic diet is a very strict system of food preparation based on a traditional, two thousand year old Japanese diet. This complicated regimen consisted of making sure the "Yin" and "Yang" properties of food were in complete balance at every meal, which meant a lot of thought and preparation went into making a meal. The mainstay of this diet is brown rice and it is considered the most balanced of all foods. So while other kids were "chowing down" on lunches of Wonder bread and peanut butter and jelly sandwiches, I was eating tofu or tempeh sandwiches with sauerkraut on whole-grain bread.

Meanwhile, at my mother's, I was fed everything "evil" according to my dad's diet – big juicy hamburgers, French fries and even milkshakes. My mother in no way approved of the way my father ate and did her very best to 'make up for it' on the days when I was in her care, encouraging me to eat red meat and all else that dad forbade. To an eight year old, this was very confusing. Add to that my summers spent with each set of grandparents – July with my dad's parents in London, England and August in Edmonton with my mum's parents – and you see why I say my diet in those days was a bit of a (pardon the expression) smorgasbord.

My dad's parents let me eat as much candy as I wanted and, for those of you who have tasted the chocolate from England, you can imagine how much I consumed! What little girl could resist? The first memory I have of obsessing about my body's shape and size is from that summer when I got back from England. I was eight. My mother looked at me in horror because I had been "fattened up" by my doting grandparents. I remember her friends commenting on how "chubby" I had become with a look of serious disappointment on their faces. Although I didn't know what chubby meant at the time, I knew it wasn't good.

When I got to my mum's parents, my well-meaning grand-mother assured my worried mother that she would fix the problem by putting me on a diet. Thus, at the tender age of eight, my eating disorder career had begun in earnest. While my grandparents ate steak and potatoes, I was fed celery sticks and tuna (without mayo of course) on Melba toast. My sweets intake was also limited and, to help me restrain myself, my granny hid the delicious cakes she made in the cellar pantry.

I didn't know it at the time but I would say now that, from that point on, I was well on my way to developing a full-blown eating disorder. Everyone in my family was obsessed with food and weight and I quickly learned to share their obsession. Being genetically predisposed to weight gain didn't help either.

I was constantly being watched in an effort to keep me from becoming fat.

And what do you think was the next thing to take me further down the slippery slope to disordered eating? Puberty, that's what. By age ten, I had developed curves and breasts and, by age twelve, I was already a very curvaceous young woman and began receiving all sorts of attention from boys and even men. The attention only fed my obsessions. I shed my so-called chubbiness quickly and was careful to remain average in size for the rest of my childhood years.

During this time, my dad moved to the United States to marry his girlfriend at the time and I was devastated by this loss. I was now living with my mum and stepfather full-time and it was not a happy situation. They fought constantly and I often found myself caught in the middle of it. I felt that I was an unwanted guest; an intruder in a home that wasn't very harmonious to begin with and that I just added one more problem to an already problematic household.

From the age of eleven onwards, I was completely boy-crazy. Boys gave me the attention and love I was missing at home and I felt as if, without their eyes on me, I would melt away into a puddle of nothingness. I felt so alone in the world and so scared when I was on my own but, when held in the adoring gaze of a young man's eyes, I felt cared for, loved, and even special.

From that point on, I went from one relationship to the next, clinging to each boyfriend as if to life itself. My eating during this time was pretty normal. I felt totally self-conscious about my body but what teenage girl doesn't? Boys seemed to like it just fine, so I figured it served its purpose.

From the age of fourteen to sixteen, I had a boyfriend who professed to want to marry me and be with me forever. You can imagine my horror when, all of a sudden, he just turned on me and told me he wanted to break up. I fell to the floor in his room, a sobbing heap begging him not to leave me. He just got angry and told me to leave. I was an absolute mess. I actually felt that my life was over.

About this time, my mother, who was forty-one, announced that she was pregnant! It was an accident, she said, but had decided to go ahead with the pregnancy anyway. Things had never been worse at home; her and my stepfather were at one other's throats constantly and I avoided being there as much as I could. I felt totally confused about why they were bringing a child into such a miserable relationship and, even though I had always wanted a sibling, I felt it was a little too late at this point.

Around this time, I became a vegetarian. My new diet invariably put my mother into a state of complete exasperation at mealtimes because she didn't want to have to make two separate meals. She soon was fed up with my non-meat-eating ways and refused to cook a separate meal for me. Instead, she gave me twenty dollars a week to go to the health food store to buy my own meat-free items.

The boy who had recently dumped me hooked up with another girl. In my sixteen-year-old mind, I deduced that he must have chosen her because she was THINNER than me. Now, my crusade to become skinny began in earnest.

I totally freaked my mother out at dinner one night when I came home from the gym and announced proudly that I had fainted while working out. I considered this a great accomplishment, an indication that I was succeeding in my weight loss goals.

I, also, read *Fit for Life* back to front, over and over again, memorizing all of the concepts of proper food combining. I carried it proudly under my arm like a bible and professed the wisdom of the words contained within to anyone who would listen. "Meat and dairy products are the foods of the devil" was my mantra.

I looked to healthy eating as a salvation from all of life's unpredictability, pain and confusion. As long as I was obsessed with what I was eating, I could ignore the emptiness, anger and hurt I was feeling inside. Planning my entire day's food before going to bed gave me a sense of the peace and order that was missing from my life; it made me feel safe and secure when nothing else around me – not my family, not my friends – could even come close to creating those feelings.

My mother gave birth to a beautiful baby girl named Ruth, after my grandmother. My stepfather, thankfully, had left. Well, didn't leave exactly; he was sort of thrown out. The day my mother went into labor, she called his work to ask him to meet her at the hospital. The person answering told her my stepfather was at "so-and-so's" house. "Who the hell is so-and-so?" my mother asked, and that was the beginning of the end.

While all of this was happening, my eating habits had gone completely off-the-wall crazy. I was following my personally devised, ultra-restrictive vegan, food-combining regimen by day followed by nightly binges on the ice cream in my mother's freezer. I'd be absolutely disgusted with myself after I'd binged – feeling like a walking slab of concrete – and would pass out on my bed with a bloated stomach, falling into a stupor that seemed closer to death than sleep. On waking, I'd chastise myself for the indulgences of the previous night, resolve to do better and basically starve myself for the entire day while simultaneously working out for two to three hours only to collapse at home after school before bingeing again the following night. I soon became addicted to herbal laxatives, which I used to purge after binges.

I was going to school and working part-time in my local health food store, evangelically educating the public about righteous eating as if I were a prophet of food standing on a mountaintop. I felt I had the key to humanity's ills and that, if I could only teach them to be healthy like me, then all would be saved.

Things at home were pretty rough at that time, also. My mother had a full-time job as a Food Editor of Canada's largest newspaper, a little baby to take care of and a teenage daughter with a life-threatening eating disorder. Oh, and she was a single mother again. I tried to hide my eating behaviors from her but she figured it out. How else can you explain three tubs of ice cream disappearing every night?

It was around this time that I suddenly developed psychological allergies to many foods and would refuse to eat them. Conveniently, I convinced myself that I was allergic to all of the foods I deemed "evil" such as white sugar, white flour, dairy, meat and a whole host of others. My many irrational allergies baffled and confused everyone around me. I used my allergies as an excuse to not eat what other people were eating and to avoid eating with others. And then, when I got home and was by myself, I would binge on all of my so-called allergy foods until I could hardly move. Then, I would take tons of laxatives to get rid of it all the next day. I continued in this manner until I was nine-teen. Finally, things started to turn around for me when I went to university.

my recovery from an eating disorder

Recovery has not come quickly or easily; eating problems are complex and extremely difficult to overcome. After all of this time in recovery (approximately eighteen years) and through my years of work as an eating disorders therapist, I no longer believe that one can completely recover from a severe eating disorder. Even after all these years of recovery, I still have a little voice inside my head that tells me life would be perfect if only I was thinner or that I would be more successful in every area of my life if, somehow, I could change the way I look.

My healing has come slowly and not without bumps and set-backs along the way. I see my recovery process as being like the act of peeling an onion, each layer representing a new discovery about myself and with each layer that is peeled back, there are tears. The tears are a way to let go of my grief and the agony that comes from understanding why I nearly killed myself through an eating disorder. The tears also represent, for me, the painful realization that roughly one-third of my young life was spent being totally obsessed with food and weight and that, try as I might, I will never be able to get those years back.

My recovery until now has consisted of a multitude of factors. In the beginning, it helped me tremendously to join a support group that emphasized emotional and spiritual growth. In this group, I learned from others who had gone further along the path to recovery than I. I learned how to eat normally and how to ask for help when I needed it. I also learned about the importance of having a spiritual connection to get me through the tough times when I was convinced I would not make it if left to my own devices. Gradually, I learned how to ask for strength to heal from the "food monster" and to receive support from – and eventually provide support to – others who were in recovery.

I have come to learn that this work is a life-long endeavor that can be done only one step at a time and that success depends on a multitude of factors, most importantly, on our own internal sense of readiness – timing is everything. Once the floodgates were opened, my life underwent a radical change. I realize now, at age 37, why I could and couldn't face certain things at different phases in my life and have great admiration and respect for how the human psyche works. I see now that, with time and experience and as I matured as an individual, I was given more to work with and gradually acquired the abilities, the means to cope. But, let me tell you, it has NOT been a fun or easy process. Nonetheless, I wouldn't trade my life for anyone else's. I am proud of who I am, who I have become and who I am becoming each and every new day. I have faced some very painful, very scary truths about my past, my family and myself and I have come out on the other side.

Every family has its secrets, its dysfunctions, its own struggles; mine is no different. The more I hear from women about their family stories in my role as therapist, the more I am confirmed in my belief that dysfunction is pervasive and that we all come from families that are, in some way, dysfunctional. This is not mere cynicism speaking but experience. I also believe that we can strive, with each passing day, to make as much sense of it all as we are able. And the good news is we are able to heal ourselves. We can let things go and, if only we choose to, we can move forward into becoming the amazing people we were meant to be.

In the chapters that follow, I intend to reveal to you what I have found to be the keys to healing from problematic relationships with food and body image. These keys are founded on a few basic principles. As a first principle, I have found it most useful to take a wholistic approach to healing and I will, therefore, outline in the following pages tried and true methods of recovery which address all aspects of our being: physical, emotional and spiritual. I have taught these methods to thousands of clients over the past decade and they have met with great success. My hope is that you, too, will benefit as much from these methods as other women have and that they provide you with both the peace and joy you are seeking.

2
types of disordered eating

In this chapter, I plan to discuss the different types of disordered eating to give you a sense of the many variations of problematic food/body image relationships that exist and that women commonly fall prey to and, thereby, help you sort out where you are on the wide spectrum of disordered eating.

Many misconceptions prevail about eating disorders and have come to make up the common fund of public knowledge about disordered eating. For most people, the two words "eating disorder" conjure up images of human skeletons, women who are on death's door whose bodies have been reduced to little more than skin and bone because of their refusal to eat, or of women who binge and purge numerous times a day and barely have any teeth left due to repeated and frequent vomiting.

All you have to do is look at the cover of any pop culture magazine to see the latest "celebrity anorexic". But the truth is much more complex than this. Though Anorexia Nervosa and Bulimia Nervosa are very serious life-threatening eating disorders that are not to be taken lightly, the fact is that these disorders affect only a very small percentage of the general female population.

Research suggests that

*   About one percent (1%) of all females have anorexia which means that about one out of every hundred young women between the ages of ten and twenty are starving themselves, sometimes to death;

*   About four percent (4%), or four out of every one hundred females, have bulimia.[1]

So what about the other 95% of the population? Keep in mind that the above statistics are probably much lower than the actual number of incidences of both anorexia and bulimia due to the many hidden sufferers who do not openly admit nor report to health professionals that they suffer from these forms of disordered eating. Even so, that still leaves a huge gap in the statistics. We know now that:

*   80-90% of women dislike the size and shape of their bodies

*   70% of women are dieting and 40% are continually gaining and losing weight

*   *One out of every two* women are on a diet

---

1   Adapted from ANRED *Statistics: How many people have eating disorders?* ANRED: Information and Resources. 28 Nov 2008. ANRED Anorexia Nervosa and Related Eating Disorders Inc.<http://www.anred.com/stats.html>.

- The majority of women *fear becoming fat more than they fear dying*[2]

I expect that the majority of you reading this fit into one or more of the above categories and stand to greatly benefit from reading the information as well as doing the exercises I put forth in the following pages. The concepts and tools I lay out in these pages have helped countless women all along the continuum of disordered eating and are general enough to apply to most situations. If, however, you suspect that you are one of those who do have a life-threatening eating disorder, I would strongly urge you to seek medical treatment immediately. Though this book may help you to a better understanding of your condition, your situation may be critical enough to warrant the one-on-one intervention of a medical practitioner with expertise in eating disorders.

The following are descriptions of the most common forms of disordered eating that I see on a day-to-day basis: Binge Eating, Anorexia Nervosa, Bulimia Nervosa and Orthorexia Nervosa. This last, I consider an important addition to the list. Though not as commonly known as its sibling conditions, it appears to be much more prevalent than in the past and on the rise due to our society's increasing focus on "healthy eating". I should mention, by the way, that it is also a condition that interests me on a personal level having suffered with it myself. To the descriptions of each of these eating disorders, I have added snippets of women's personal stories as illustration.

---

2   Speaking as a psychotherapist who has worked with thousands of women with various forms of disordered eating for over a decade, I would say that at least 85% of my clients struggling with food and body image issues are not anorexic or bulimic, nor are their eating disorders life-threatening. For the most part these women are struggling with bouts of overeating, yo-yo dieting involving 10-30 pound weight gains and losses, general discomfort with their bodies, and a preoccupation with food, weight, and the size and shape of their bodies.

binge eating/compulsive eating

I find that the vast majority of women I work with struggle with binge eating, otherwise known as compulsive overeating. Going on the latest fad diet often precipitates binge eating. Women suffering from binge eating often fall through the cracks of the mental health system because their disorder isn't viewed as being "serious" enough for government-funded treatment. These women are viewed by the system as not being "medically compromised" and as still able to function to a reasonably high standard. Since most women with eating problems fall into this category, a significant portion of women suffering from binge eating go without the help and support they need to treat their disorder.

A study reported in *Drugs and Therapy Perspectives* (15(5): 7-10, March 13, 2000) indicates that 30% of women in the United States who seek treatment to lose weight have binge eating disorder. In other studies, up to 2% – or one to two million adults in the U.S. alone – have problems with binge eating. Once again, keep in mind that these statistics are probably much lower than actual numbers because many people with disordered eating issues do not self-report due to the shame they feel.

While I work with all types of disordered eating, I would say that around 85% of the women who come to me for help are binge eaters or compulsive overeaters. The following is a list of the diagnostic criteria for "Binge Eating Disorder" as it appears in the DSM-IV, Diagnostic and Statistical Manual of Mental Disorders:

Diagnostic Criteria: Binge Eating Disorder

1. Recurrent episodes of binge eating. An episode is characterized by:

   - Eating a larger amount of food than normal during a short period of time (within any two hour period)

   - Lack of control over eating during the binge episode (i.e. the feeling that one cannot stop eating).

2. Binge eating episodes are associated with three or more of the following:

   - Eating until feeling uncomfortably full

   - Eating large amounts of food when not physically hungry

   - Eating much more rapidly than normal

   - Eating alone because you are embarrassed by how much you're eating

   - Feeling disgusted, depressed, or guilty after overeating

3. Marked distress regarding binge eating is present

4. Binge eating occurs, on average, at least 2 days a week for six months

5. Binge eating is not associated with the regular use of inappropriate compensatory behavior (i.e. purging, excessive ex-

ercise, etc.) and does not occur exclusively during the course of bulimia nervosa or anorexia nervosa.

The following snippets from women's experiences of binge eating behaviours come from the website: www.something-fishy.org. They echo what I hear every day in my office from clients struggling with compulsive overeating.

I have good days and I have bad days! If I am alone in the house, that is my worst. I can eat cookies, ice cream, cereal, etc. – whatever is good and full of fat. If my husband is home, I sneak food. When he goes to get the mail, I stuff a couple of cookies in my mouth and, when he gets back, the proof is gone! I act like I have not eaten all day, then suggest we go to dinner or to Dairy Queen when really I have been pounding down the goodies all day. This has been going on for years, even before I was married. I have gone up & down in weight so much. I can't stop these things I do to myself. I have tried all diets & pills (which I am sorry for taking because of my problems due to the new diet drugs!). I have tried to get a tummy tuck. I had a breast reduction. I take pills like No Doz but these things only work for so long. Then I start eating a lot again.

There is never a time that I am not consumed with food. I'm either thinking about food or eating. I work out regularly and am quite busy, so I appear to everyone else to be chunky rather than obese. No one has any idea how much food I eat or how much I think about eating. I eat normally in front of people and sneak the rest. I have driven (by myself, of course) to a fast food restaurant, ordered a large cheeseburger, fries and a drink, eaten the entire meal in less than 5 minutes,

*then driven directly to a different fast food restaurant
and ordered more. I will purposefully wrap all of the
containers and bags up as small as I can and stop where
no one knows me and throw the evidence away. I even
sneak food into the bathroom at home, turn the fan
on so no one can hear the food wrappers rattling and
binge. I eat until I feel ill. Many times if I am prevent-
ed from eating, like if someone comes over unexpectedly,
I feel extremely angry and anxious. I have no idea why
this is happening to me and feel powerless to stop this
madness.*

*To me, compulsive overeating is a disease where a per-
son has no control over their food intake. It's a constant
eating, a wanting for more and more. You can't get
enough, sort of like a junkie looking for the next high.
That is my relationship with food. And I have no control. I consider myself intelligent, well schooled in many
areas. I know what types of things I should be eating to
maintain a healthy lifestyle but I just can't do it. I don't
understand why I can't. I'll eat because I'm bored, lone-
ly, depressed, happy, stressed out, etc. And I don't know
when to stop. However, when I do stop, I feel horrible.
So stuffed I can barely move. If I continue on this path
of destruction, I will not live very much longer.*

anorexia nervosa

The following are the diagnostic criteria for Anorexia Nervosa as it appears in the DSM-IV, Diagnostic and Statistical Manual of Mental Disorders:

Diagnostic Criteria: Anorexia Nervosa

1. Refusal to maintain body weight at or above a minimally normal weight for age and height (e.g. weight loss leading to maintenance of body weight less than 85% of that expected; or failure to make expected weight gain during period of growth, leading to body weight less than 85% of that expected).

2. Intense fear of gaining weight or becoming fat even though underweight.

3. Disturbance in the way in which one's body weight or shape is experienced, undue influence of body weight or shape on self-evaluation, or denial of the seriousness of the current low body weight.

4. In postmenarcheal females, amenorrhea, (i.e. the absence of at least three consecutive menstrual cycles).

Restricting Type
During the current episode of Anorexia Nervosa, the person has not regularly engaged in binge eating or purging behaviour (i.e. self-induced vomiting or the misuse of laxatives, diuretics or enemas).

Binge-Eating/Purging Type
During the current episode of Anorexia Nervosa, the person has regularly engaged in binge eating or purging behavior (i.e.

self-induced vomiting or the misuse of laxatives, diuretics, or enemas).

Here are snippets from the story of a 19-year-old woman with anorexia who kindly sent me the following to help with this book.

My struggle with anorexia began when I was twelve and a half years old. I cannot remember clearly the first time I decided, sitting amongst the coats in the cloakroom staring at my lunch, that the answer to life's problems was to throw it away, or why a few days later it seemed like the right thing to do to repeat the pattern, and spend the afternoon with the strangely pleasant feeling of hunger tapping away inside me. I thought that it would just be the once, but of course it never is. I had no idea that that day marked a turning point in my life: that throwing my lunch away one day because I felt miserable would take me down the road to hell and back. Six years ago I never imagined I would become addicted to the hunger that slowly crept into my life; and two years ago I never believed I'd escape the grip of that hunger, the anorexia, that took over my life.

I'm the stereotype of anorexics: a white, middle class, well educated young girl, my parents still married at that point. I'd just begun high school that September, giving me a freedom with food not experienced in primary school where we ate what was given to us at lunch. Moving schools coincided with hitting puberty and suddenly having pimples, greasier hair and inevitable weight gain. I'd never been aware of my weight before, or my looks to a great extent. Now, I just wanted to fit in with everyone else but felt so much more ugly and unfashionable; and then I started to feel fat. So I suppose these were the things that contributed to the initial decision to not eat my lunch. And I found that doing so gave me power over my ugly body and my life. I was in control.

It didn't take long for it to become a regular habit. Sometimes friends succeeded in coaxing me to eat my lunch so breakfast got smaller until I threw it away on my way to school. I became conscious of whatever I ate, hating every mouthful of the dinner that I had to eat, not wanting anyone at home to become suspicious. For the next six months or so I would sometimes 'come to my senses' and eat normally for a few days, but then I'd feel guilty and eat as little as possible for the next few days. When my parents separated that summer, the instability at home increased. Now I couldn't possibly eat, I told myself.

I really didn't deserve food now. The anorexic voices worsened, feeding on my unhappiness. I obsessed more and more over my weight, worrying if it went up, seeing it as an achievement when some months my period wouldn't arrive because my weight had dropped a little. Due to the fact that I was growing, I never lost much weight during the next two years of this pattern, so my parents didn't catch onto what I was doing.

I crashed quickly; buckling under the pressure I put myself under to maintain the good grades I was getting. I spent all my free time studying or reading alone in my room, hiding from the world. This created the perfect condition for the anorexia to grow on and, within a matter of weeks, I was down a stone. Diet pills became a necessity and I'd take them at every non-existent meal, then 10 times the recommended amount at 'dinner' as punishment for giving into cravings for maybe a bread roll or some soup. Everyone knew I was slipping, but I refused their help because this was all I wanted more than anything, to starve myself away. I seemed to want the voice that was driving me towards hell, to thrive on the hunger that had become my closest friend and felt success when my weight dropped lower than ever.

bulimia nervosa

Here are the diagnostic criteria for Bulimia Nervosa as it appears in the DSM-IV, Diagnostic and Statistical Manual of Mental Disorders:

Diagnostic Criteria: Bulimia Nervosa

1. Recurrent episodes of binge eating. An episode of binge eating is characterized by both of the following:

   - Eating, in a discrete period of time (e.g., within any 2-hour period), an amount of food that is definitely larger than most people would eat during a similar period of time and under similar circumstances.

   - A sense of lack of control over eating during the episode (e.g., a feeling that one cannot stop eating or control what or how much one is eating)

2. Recurrent inappropriate compensatory behavior in order to prevent weight gain, such as self-induced vomiting; misuse of laxatives, diuretics, enemas, or other medications; fasting or excessive exercise.

3. The binge eating and inappropriate compensatory behaviors both occur, on average, at least twice a week for 3 months.

4. Self-evaluation is unduly influenced by body shape and weight.

5. The disturbance does not occur exclusively during episodes of Anorexia Nervosa.

Purging Type
During the current episode of Bulimia Nervosa, the person has regularly engaged in self-induced vomiting or the misuse of laxatives, diuretics or enemas.

Non-purging Type
During the current episode of Bulimia Nervosa, the person has used other inappropriate compensatory behaviours such as fasting or excessive exercise, but has not regularly engaged in self-induced vomiting or the misuse of laxatives, diuretics or enemas.

Here are snippets of stories from a teenager and a 23-year-old with bulimia who kindly sent me the following to help with this book. I have changed the names of the people in their stories to protect their anonymity:

I developed bulimia when I was fifteen years old. I had struggled with my weight since I was a child. When I began purging I thought I could stop as soon as I reached my goal weight, but this was surely not the case. Instead, bulimia nervosa ruled my life.

I began binging and purging daily. I was losing weight so rapidly that my mom had to buy me new clothes every other weekend. My mother would get upset because food would turn up missing because of my constant binging. I would lie every night and tell her that I was going to take a shower, but instead I would purge.

Everything seemed to be a lie. A year went by and I got down to a hundred and eleven pounds. I think I lost all aspects of my identity. I was no longer living as Judy; I was simply a girl with bulimia. This disease spoke for me, lied for me, and lived for me. I could think of nothing else but getting food, eating it and, more importantly, getting rid of it. I began throwing up in my bedroom so I would not be in the bathroom so long. I was afraid of getting caught.

I hit rock bottom with my eating disorder the day I got a phone call from Lucy's mother. She was a friend of mine who also had bulimia. Her mother told me that Lucy was in the hospital because her esophagus nearly ruptured. I could not breathe while I was hearing this. My mind was overloaded with thoughts that I could lose my best friend, or that I could die at any moment from heart failure due to an electrolyte imbalance.

After a few weeks of living away the bulimia became really bad again. I began missing lectures to binge. I'd lock myself away for days and just binge and vomit. I wasted money and time.

I felt ill and useless. I felt like I was wasting myself. I would cancel meeting friends and doing things because of the bulimia. Once I got into the mood for a binge, nothing would stop me. Again I was being controlled by the eating disorder. I felt like giving up on everything. I often couldn't face doing work so I would just binge. Sometimes I would take laxatives, which would make me feel really ill and in pain.

Throughout the last years of my eating disorder, I have made regular visits to the dentist and doctor. I have had one tooth out due to the many infections I'd get in my mouth from vomiting all the time. Once, my jaw locked from an infection. I sunk to the lowest of the low. Some of the things I did I could never tell, I am so ashamed.

orthorexia nervosa

Steven Bratman, M.D., coined the term "orthorexia nervosa" in 1997 from the Greek word *ortho* – which means " straight, correct and true " – in order to distinguish this eating disorder from the better-known anorexia nervosa. In his book, *Orthorexia: Health Food Junkies Overcoming the Obsession with Healthful Eating*, Dr. Bratman describes orthorexia as a disease in which people fixate on eating healthy food.

At this time, orthorexia is not categorized in the DSMIV as an actual eating disorder but many mental health professionals consider it a sub-clinical form of an eating disorder. Statistics on orthorexia are hard to pin down because it's such a new concept. In time, I expect we'll be hearing a lot more about this disorder and will learn more not only about the condition itself but also about the many thousands of people who, in my estimation, are being affected by this illness.

Dr. Bratman states that orthorexia is similar to anorexia and bulimia with this one difference: "Whereas the bulimic and anorexic focus on the quantity of food, the orthorexic fixates on its quality."

Although I have experienced elements of all of the above types of disordered eating, I would say that most of my behaviors around food fall into the orthorexic category. For evidence of this, just go back and read my story at the beginning of the book.

I see this type of disordered eating especially on the rise where I live on the West Coast. Everyone knows the stereotype of the West Coast dwellers commonly referred to as "granolas" with their obsessively healthy lifestyle and their restrictive good-for-you diets. While this description doesn't apply to everyone who lives in these parts, it has become something of a stereotype for a reason. It fairly describes the lifestyle of a not insignificant portion of the population in these parts. Sometimes, it seems there exists an inordinate focus on being fit, outdoorsy and healthy in body, mind and spirit. In fact, that's precisely why I moved out here in the first place.

While being healthy is a great idea, like any other, it can in practice be taken to extremes, can overtake one's life and can turn into a habit that is decidedly not healthy. I think the greatest example of this is what I see happening in the so-called "raw food" movement. Indeed, I was "all raw" myself for five months! I know a lot of people here who are strict raw-food vegans who won't eat anything cooked, believing as they do that cooked food is bad for you.

Among these raw food and health food types, it is not uncommon to find extremely zealous and self-righteous people. It seems to me that, for many, raw food has become a sort of cult-like belief and that belonging to the cult, by necessity, means cutting yourself off from everyone who eats normally, that is, people who eat cooked food. As a result, there is not much sharing of meals with family and friends; at least not those who don't share your food philosophy, and you can say a fond farewell to restaurants and most other forms of social dining. The choice to be a "raw foodist" has very profound social implications, indeed.

When I was eating all raw, I felt righteous and superior to others and couldn't understand why other people were "killing themselves" by eating inferior cooked food. I did feel great physically and had lots of energy but my social life totally sucked and I couldn't see how I was using my diet to separate myself from my fellow human beings. My arrogance, rigidity and self-righteousness made it impossible for me to appreciate the social hurt my eating habits were causing me. Looking back, I can't imagine that I was much fun to be around. Little wonder, I spent much of my time eating alone during that period of my life.

If you think, based on what you've read here, that you may be suffering from orthorexia, I strongly suggest you read Steven Bratman's book. It's a wonderful resource full of invaluable information for the orthorexia sufferer. There is little doubt in my mind that this gem of a book has already helped countless people to rid themselves of their health food obsessions and return to the human fold.

3
why diets don't work

I've decided to start the recovery portion of this book by discussing "Why Diets Don't Work". If my many years of practice have taught me anything, it's that the habit of dieting is at the root of most, if not all, dysfunctional eating. Moreover, it's a well-known fact that dieting is the major precursor to serious eating disorders such as anorexia and bulimia nervosa, which are extremely dangerous and life threatening.

In this chapter, I will start by giving you some statistics and facts about dieting and why it's so dangerous. After that, I will share some of my thoughts based on my experience working with women with eating disorders about why it is we keep on dieting. We'll also talk about who is profiting most from this often highly injurious and destructive habit. Finally, I'll offer a detailed outline of what happens to us physiologically when we diet and how this sets up a self-perpetuating cycle of defeat.

In the second part of this chapter, I'm going to give you an opportunity, through some simple exercises, to delve into your own history of dieting, food obsession, weight loss and weight gain with the hope of opening your mind to some healthier alternatives to dieting. I chose to take this approach as a psychotherapist because I have found that true, lasting change only comes about when we do our own personal work. It's not enough to simply listen to someone else's story or to some expert, such as myself, pontificating on the dangers of dieting. We need to take the advice and the knowledge received and apply them to our own experience. This can only be done once we've gone far enough below the surface to find the root causes of our problematic relationship to food and body image.

In a sense, I'm giving you the opportunity to do some of your own therapy right now, right here, within the pages of this book. You may find that you need outside help at certain points as these exercises may stir up a lot of emotions and recall memories of unfinished and unresolved business from your past. If this happens, I strongly suggest that you see a psycho-therapist in person for individual sessions to help move you through these areas of difficulty and challenge.

For these hands-on exercises, you're welcome to use the pages of this book but you may need additional paper on which to record your answers. And, of course, you'll need a pen; pos-sibly, a handful of pens. Even better, you could keep a journal dedicated to doing the exercises throughout this book so that you can keep track of your progress as you go along and have something to refer back to when needed.

I will also share with you a funny, inspirational story of a re-covered dieter that you will, in all probability, be able to relate to and from which, I hope, you'll be able to gain some wisdom. Lastly, I will share some very practical and useful information about what "normal eating" looks like so that, immediately upon reading this first of our recovery chapters, you can start the process of transforming how you relate to food. I hope you find this experience informative, enlightening and helpful in your journey to finding peace with food and your body.

a few dieting facts

- An astonishing 50% of young girls in Canada begin dieting before the age of nine; 81% of 10-year olds diet and at least 46% of 9 year olds restrict their eating.

- In the U.S., 7-17 year olds are the heaviest users of diet pills.

- 71% of adolescent girls want to be thinner despite the fact that only a small proportion of young girls are clinically overweight.

- The fear of fat is so overwhelming that young girls have indicated in surveys that they are more afraid of becoming fat than they are of cancer, nuclear war or losing their parents.

dieting leads to serious eating disorders

- 90% of those people diagnosed with an eating disorder are female.

- Eating disorders are now the third most common chronic illness in adolescent girls.

- Eating disorders have the highest mortality rate of any mental illness.

- While the most common age of onset is between 14 and 25 years of age, eating disorders can occur within a wide range of ages and are increasingly seen in children as young as 10 years of age.

- The death rate associated with anorexia nervosa alone is more than 12 times higher than the overall death rate among young women in the general population.

- It is estimated that a staggering 3% of women will be affected by eating disorders in their lifetime.

what really happens when we diet?

How we diet	What really happens
By skipping meals or decreasing calories	Lowers metabolism so we store fat more easily from fewer calories
	The brain's and muscle's demand for fuel causes rebound "munchies", usually for high fat and high sugar items
	Poor attention span, irritability, fatigue
	Muscle tissue may be lost
By eliminating starchy foods (i.e. Atkins Diet)	Your body loses its best source of stable energy, and you'll likely feel moody and tired
	You'll end up eating higher fat and sugary foods to satisfy munchies

How we diet	What really happens
By going on preplanned meal replacement diet or liquid diet	You have a 95% chance of regaining any weight you lose in 1-2 years You give away control to the plan which lowers your self-esteem You often lose muscle mass along with fat which lowers your metabolism, making it easier to store fat on fewer calories Habits are replaced temporarily, not changed permanently It's expensive! (In 1990, the diet industry posted an excess of $32 BILLION. Imagine what it is now!)
By fasting	Most of weight loss is water Muscle mass decreases which lowers metabolism- leads to weight gain Can be medically dangerous for some
To be slim	Slimness is temporary. Over the long run, 95% of dieters regain the weight. Many women get fatter so they diet again with similar poor results. This is called diet cycling and can lead to obesity

How we diet	What really happens
To be healthier	Diet cycling increases health risks more than being overweight
	There is no evidence that being fat is unhealthy. There is evidence to show that being too thin is unhealthy
	Most dieting decreases our muscle mass. Muscles are needed for good health.
	Many diets are unhealthy. Your body and mind don't run well when you restrict calories. Dieting makes you cranky and obsessed with food. This feels like a failure, but is just a physiological response and has nothing at all to do with willpower
To be more attractive	What attracts you to someone else? Do you want your friends to like you for your body or who you are? What are long-term relationships based upon? If you are dieting, are you any fun to be around?

Adapted from material provided by The British Columbia Ministry of Health and Ministry Responsible for Seniors.

top 10 reasons to give up dieting

1. **Diets don't work.** Even if you lose weight, you will probably gain it all back and you might gain back more than you lost.

2. **Diets are expensive.** If you didn't buy special diet products, you could save enough to get new clothes, which would improve your outlook and your appearance right now.

3. **Diets are boring.** People on diets talk and think about food and practically nothing else. There's a lot more to life than food.

4. **Diets don't necessarily improve your health.** Like weight loss, health improvement is temporary. Dieting can actually cause health problems.

5. **Diets don't make you beautiful.** Very few people will ever look like models. Glamour is a look not a size. You don't have to be thin to be attractive.

6. **Diets are not sexy.** If you want to be more attractive, take care of your body and your appearance. Feeling healthy makes you look your best.

7. **Diets can turn into life-threatening eating disorders.** The obsession to be thin can lead to anorexia, bulimia, bingeing and compulsive exercising.

8. **Diets can make you afraid of food.** Food nourishes and comforts us and gives us pleasure. Dieting can make food seem like your enemy and can deprive you of all the positives about food.

9. **Diets can rob you of energy.** If you want to live a full and active life, you need good nutrition and enough food to meet your body's needs.

And the number one reason to give up dieting is...

10. **Learning to love and accept yourself** just as you are will give you self-confidence, better health and a sense of well-being that will last a lifetime.

Adapted from the 1994 Council on Size and Weight Discrimination, Inc.

Now that I've given you some information about dieting and why it's a complete waste of your time, energy and money, it's time to shift our focus to YOU. Let me begin by guiding you in doing some of the personal reflection that will help you to begin to let go of the dieting mentality permanently.

I am going to ask you three, apparently simple, questions to begin this process. Don't rip yourself off by writing the short, obvious answers to what may appear to be simple questions. I invite you to really meditate on each question and take as much time as you need to fully answer them.

Do some soul-searching and answer each question as thoroughly and honestly as you are able, particularly the last one. When you think you're done, dig a little deeper. Continue digging until you feel you've gotten to the bottom of things, until you're convinced you've told the whole truth and nothing but the truth.

Remember: you're doing this for you and no one else. You owe it to yourself to spend time reflecting on this aspect of your life that has caused you so much grief.

How many diets have you been on in your life?

Have any of them worked over the long-term for you?

Why do you diet?

Now, draw a large circle on this page. Turn the circle into a "pie" chart by dividing it into sections. Section off how much of your time on any given day is taken up thinking about food, weight and how you look. Give it a percentage.

If you could wave a magic wand and make this focus on food, weight and how you look disappear completely, just think what you could accomplish with all the time you've gained? List here all the interests you might pursue, the activities you might engage in, the basic chores you might stop neglecting and finally get done in your day.

List all of the things you've always dreamed of doing but have never found the time for.

Write until you have exhausted all possibilities.

Now, I want you to close your eyes for a minute, take in some deep breaths and imagine yourself doing those things you've written on your list. How do you feel inside? On this page, either draw an image of that feeling or write it out in words. Refer to this often as you continue through this book.

Next, I invite you take a break from writing and self-reflection, sit back, relax and read a personal story of a recovering dieter. It's called *Fat Like Me* and was written by Terry Poulton, author of *No Fat Chicks: How Big Business Profits by Making Women Hate Their Bodies – And How to Fight Back.* This is a fabulous book and I highly recommend you pick up a copy and read it cover to cover.

There's something only Oprah Winfrey and I know from actual experience: hell is having to show up fat when the whole country knows you're supposed to be thin.

Oprah handled it by wailing to her diary about how disgusted she was with herself. I tried something a little goofier during the winter of 1983, while regaining the 65 pounds Chatelaine readers had watched me whittle away during an arduous six-month stint when I practically camped in a gym crunching carrot sticks and little else. From Truro to Temiscaming to Tofino, my "Chronicles of the Incredible Shrinking Terry" attracted fan letters and resulted in my photos being plastered on fridge doors and gym walls. After a lifetime as a wall-flower, I was a hero to every woman who ever longed to be slim.

And then, my pet albatross came flapping back to its longtime roost (just as these tenacious birds do to most dieters). I was a freelance magazine writer in media-savvy Toronto, where all my colleagues knew to the pound what I was supposed to weigh. As I rapidly re-inflated, I tried toiling as much as possible by phone and memo but, eventually, I had to show up for editorial meetings. That's when I hatched a gambit worthy of Lucy Ricardo at her ditziest. Instead of wearing a warm winter coat, I flung a big green cape over my pre-diet raincoat. Then, whenever I made an entrance, I dramatically swirled the cape off and remained hidden (I hoped) inside my raincoat. If any of my colleagues caught on, they were kind enough not to squeal.

Thirteen years later, I can finally laugh at my transparent ply instead of cringing from the sense of failure that dogged me from childhood until very recently. I now realize that I sacrificed too many precious years trying to obey a virtual commandment I didn't really believe: Women Must Be Thin. Even while taking a very public bow for losing a third of my body weight, I sensed that I was betraying myself and those I'd influenced into blind conformity. "No one can make you feel inferior without your consent," Eleanor Roosevelt once wrote. Somewhere inside, I knew I had given my consent to inferior treatment, not only for overweight women, but for everyone who embodies something-anything-our society despises. This sank in only after many subsequent spins on the diet carousel and even a stomach-stapling operation. When I finally understood it, I began achieving what I really wanted all along: respect, from myself and from others.

What I hoped would be my "diet to end all diets" was set in motion by Chatelaine editors who knew about my Herculean, totally typical, lifelong battle with excess weight. Although I was never a compulsive binger eater, I did lead a sedentary life. That, plus decades of yo-yo weight levels, slowed my metabolism and strip-mined my body of lean muscle tissue. Like many of the estimated 29% of overweight Canadian women-and the 60% who are trying to lose weight-I'd been on dozens of diets, and lost and regained hundreds of pounds.

After a lucky start as a precocious, pretty and beloved child growing up in Alberta, I lost my golden-girl status when I became fat in pre-pubescence. None of my good qualities seemed to count anymore, as praise and friendship were replaced by taunts and ostracism. Although pictures of me as a teenager don't look all that bad, I felt like a monster. By the time I reached my 20s, bag-of-bones Twiggy had replaced curvy Marilyn Monroe as the reigning standard of beauty. I was so determined to conform to the increasingly narrow parameters of acceptability that, by my 30s, I had tried even such extreme measures as noxious daily injections (which compelled me to crave raw meat) and consuming nothing but liquid protein for five months a la Oprah and with even worse results, as I wound up losing my gallbladder.

Enter my editorial chums at Chatelaine. They would pick up the tab for sending me to nutritional, fitness and psychological counseling if I would promise to lose 65 pounds and write about my experiences along the way.

It seemed like every woman's dream. After all, who hasn't suffered from the "if only" syndrome? If only I were like Oprah, we think, and had the money for a personal chef and trainer, plus a free fitness center in which to go for the burn…then I could get in shape and my life would be perfect. Seduced by my "if only" dream, I had no idea I was beginning the toughest and lone-

liest time of my life, in which I'd force-march myself through my own private boot camp trying to meet the scariest deadline of my career.

At first, the pounds came off steadily as I trudged and ached my way along, remaining mostly faithful to my prudent eating and exercising plan. If I just kept on losing over 10 pounds a month, I'd have it made. But I fell off the wagon one month while traveling and hit a plateau during another. Shortly after the halfway point, a fear that was bubbling below my consciousness burst into full-blown terror. I still had 40 pounds to lose and only three months until the deadline. I was in big trouble.

What no one understood back then was how implacably the human body is programmed to fight when it perceives famine conditions such as I had imposed upon myself during and before the Chatelaine diet. The less I ate and the more I pushed my body to expend energy, the more stubbornly it slowed my metabolism. In other words, it wasn't just pigging out but also starving that had contributed to my excess body fat. If I were a cavewoman who couldn't find food, this would have saved my life. Instead, with all of Canada watching, I was headed for the worst failure of my life.

Defeat or drastic measures were my only options, and I chose the latter. To be closer to the suburban fitness center, which was 32 kilometers from my home, I walked out on the man I had been planning to marry, promising to return as soon as I reached my goal. Three weeks later, I found another woman had taken my place.

Meanwhile, I was alone in a shabby apartment with nothing but a single chair and a mattress on the floor. In the kitchen, I kept only skim milk and coffee. My nutritionist had forbidden caffeine but without it, I had no energy at all. To beat the crowd, I would hit the gym every morning at about 6:30 and work out for at least an hour amid blatantly disapproving stares from skinny patrons. Exhausted and breathless, I would then shower, dress, stumble to my car and race to Toronto to work on writing projects. I had no time for family, friends or anything but the all-consuming need to hit my deadline.

At the end of days during which I often ate as few as half of my prescribed 1,000-1,2000 calories, I would zip back to the gym, repeat my morning's workout and then swim 22 laps in the Olympic-size pool. Sometimes sleep brought blessed oblivion afterward; sometimes I tossed all night. The following day, and the day after that, I would do it all again. Then I would write another segment of my Chatelaine series in the sunny positive style that hid my tattered pride. "Because my diet and exercising have brought such good results", I trilled in a typical prevarication, "my general attitude and self-image have improved tremendously and I'm almost constantly euphoric."

Meanwhile, another magazine assigned me a feature story on a woman whose obsession with becoming thin actually killed her when diuretics and appetite-suppressing drugs fatally damaged her heart. As I listened to the testimony at her inquest and realized that her struggles were only slightly more desperate than mine, I felt frightened about the possible consequences of my regimen. Even worse was a suspicion that in my effort to get slim, I was squandering the gift of just being alive. If I hadn't been so publicly committed to my diet, I would have quit. Instead, I persevered.

And then, in June of 1982, there I was, beaming on the cover of Chatelaine, 65 pounds lighter and suddenly a media star. As I drifted from microphone to camera, I tried to ignore a sense of turmoil that grew with every compliment that revealed the contempt in which I had previously been held. Keep smiling, I remember telling myself. You've won. You're finally giving them what they demanded. They're finally giving you what you were really hungry for: not food, but acceptance.

I gradually sensed there was something ugly about this admiration. Where were these people before I bought their approval? Why couldn't they see I was the same worthwhile person I had always been?

Anger, ambivalence and disappointment drove me back to comfort food, a sedentary life and the inevitable consequences: regained weight and renewed despair. On the face of things, I was a successful columnist for a major newspaper, but inside, I felt as scorned as ever.

Eight years after my Chatelaine triumph, I had fallen into the life of a near-hermit. I moved to Louisville, KY, without really understanding what compelled me. Ostensibly, it was to be near my sister, her three grown children and, especially, my 2-year-old godson. I'd never married or had children–I'd put my life on hold until I could be thin.

When a literary agent suggested I write a book about being fat in a society that demands thin, I hesitated. But as I did some serious research, I found the key that unlocked the psychological prison in which I had wasted 40 years.

The key is money-money in the pocket of those who sell wannabe waifs an array of weight-loss services worth an estimated $300 billion annually in Canada alone. In pursuit of this profit, our society has been brainwashed with the idea that attractiveness equals the emaciated forms we see on-screen and in magazines.

When I understood how this scam worked, anger and outrage finally ousted the shame. At the same time, I realized that it was not gluttony but frantic dieting that had kept me fat-and this liberated me from a lifetime of obsession and guilt.

My attitude toward how I treat my body has been transformed. I now freely choose when to work out and what I eat. I've probably lost 30 pounds, but I promised myself never to step on a scale again. When I gaze at my reflection today, whether in a mirror or in other people's eyes, I no longer see the grotesque, fun-house distortion that tormented me for so long. Instead, I see what I always wanted to see: a contented, self-respecting, normal person. I'm not slender, but neither is the average North American woman, especially in middle age. Nor am I "proud to be fat", as some advocates for the laudable size-acceptance movement declare. I am just me. And it's finally enough."

Now, on the next page, I'd like you to do the following exercise....

If you were to throw away everything you've ever learned about food, weight and body image from outside sources and pretend that you had all the answers within yourself to make peace with food and your body, what would you do?

Write a list of goals for yourself.

Write it out in detail and, again, don't stop until you've made your list of goals as complete as it can be.

Choose one goal from your list and now make a list of steps you might take over the next week in order to reach or, at least, begin to approach that goal.

Commit to taking at least one action step this week and when you've accomplished it, write about how it felt below:

4
mindful eating

In this chapter, I will share with you everything I know about mindful eating. We'll start with a mindful eating exercise, followed by a discussion of how mindful eating can become an incredibly powerful tool in helping you to find peace with food and your body. The remainder of the chapter will focus on what I believe are the five major roadblocks to eating mindfully. I will lead you through several hands-on exercises designed to assist you to identify your own personal roadblocks and how you can move past them to begin eating with mindful awareness and a sense of peace and well-being.

For these exercises, you will be doing a lot of writing so get out your favourite pen. You will also need one fresh apple slice for the first exercise. So, go cut up an apple and bring a slice back to where you're sitting so we can get started.

I'll wait here....

Done? Okay, now, I will lead you through a mindful eating exercise. Read through the entire exercise then stop and take the time to perform it. Perform the exercise slowly, meditatively, mindfully. Make it last.

Closing your eyes, take a bite of your apple slice. Do not begin chewing just yet but let the apple sit on your tongue.

Clear your mind of all distracting thoughts, focusing all your thought solely on the apple. Notice anything that comes to mind about the apple's taste, texture, temperature and any sensations in your mouth being aroused by the apple.

Now, begin chewing the apple. Chew slowly, observing what it feels and tastes like to bite into the apple. It's normal that your mind will tend to wander off. If you notice you're paying more attention to your thoughts and not the act of chewing, just let go of the thought for the moment and come back to the chewing. Notice each tiny movement of your jaw and mentally record all the sensations that you're experiencing.

In these moments, you may find yourself wanting to swallow the apple. Try to resist, putting off swallowing to the last possible moment. Mindful eating is not a race. Now, see if you can stay present and notice the subtle transition from chewing to swallowing. As you prepare to swallow the apple, try to follow it moving toward the back of your tongue and into your throat. Finally swallow the apple, following it until you can no longer feel any sensation of the food remaining.

Take a deep breath and exhale.[1]

---

1   Adapted from *Mastering the Mindful Meal* by Stephanie Vangsness, R.D., L.D.N., C.N.S.D.

Having performed the exercise, take a few minutes here to write down all the sensations, both physical and emotional, that you experienced while doing the exercise.

Were there any surprises? If so, what were they?

Mindfulness practice helps us bring all of our awareness to the here and now, focusing on the sensations in our bodies and our breathing, instead of letting it slip away while thinking about the past or the future or anything else that isn't real in this moment.

According to the Buddhists who invented mindfulness practice, we have three states of mind.

The Reasonable Mind
This is your rational, thinking, logical mind. It is the part of you that plans and evaluates things logically.

The Emotional Mind
You know you are in the grips of your emotional mind when you do or say things without thinking them through first (i.e. your emotions influence and control your thinking and your behavior).

The Wise Mind
This is the state you are in when the emotional mind and reasonable mind are working together harmoniously. Your wise mind can know and experience the truth. It is quiet. You feel centered when you're there. You feel peaceful.

The main goal of practicing mindfulness on a regular basis is to achieve the "wise mind" state as often as possible. Mindful eating is a skill which can be learned just like any other and practiced when you want to slow down, get centered and be in the moment with the food in front of you. While it may seem awkward and difficult at first, with consistent practice, applying mindfulness to our eating becomes second nature.[2]

2   Linehan, M. *Skills Training Manual for Treating Borderline Personality Disorder*. New York: Guilford Press, 1993.

Eating mindfully means eating with awareness – not so much awareness of what foods are on your plate but, rather, awareness of the experience of eating. Mindful eating is being present, moment-by-moment, for each sensation that happens during eating, that is, chewing, tasting and swallowing.

If you've ever practiced mindfulness in any way – as meditation, relaxation or breathing exercises, for example – you are familiar with how readily our minds tend to wander and you can appreciate the discipline required to keep it from wandering.

The same thing happens when we eat as performing any other activity. When you begin to practice mindful eating, it is important to remember not to judge yourself when your mind drifts off. Instead, just keep returning to the awareness of the food in front of you: the smell, texture, taste, chew, bite or swallow.

I'd like you to read what one of the most esteemed "gurus" of mindfulness, Jon Kabat-Zinn, has to say about mindfulness and eating. The following excerpt is taken from his book, *Coming to Our Senses: Healing Ourselves and the World Through Mindfulness.*

> *After breathing, eating is just about as basic as it gets for living organisms. We cannot sustain ourselves without eating, and the drives to satisfy that daily need for sustenance, in particular hunger and thirst, along with the discrimination of taste, which in the wild reduced the chances of poisoning ourselves out of desperation when hungry or thirsty, require daily satisfaction.*

> *In hunting-and-gathering societies, almost all the energy of every able-bodied person went into procuring food. In agricultural societies, where the majority*

of food is grown and raised rather than hunted and gathered, a huge amount of energy in the society still goes into food production. Nevertheless, agriculture and the raising of animals over time, at least in locations where the environment was conducive to it, provided surpluses of food that allowed for a growing complexity within social groups, the appearance of cities and civil society, wherein not everybody devoted their energies to food production or distribution even though everybody in the society has to eat to stay alive. This trend has obviously continued and has become even more the case in industrial and post-industrial societies. Thus, our relationship to food over the past ten thousand years has changed dramatically, including the ease of procurement, preservation, storage, distribution, and varieties of food available to us, its quality and nutritive value, and the ubiquity of it. From that have arisen many ways in which we who do not grow or catch our own food, take both food and eating for granted, and we live very far from the basic need to find food when it is scarce or difficult to procure.

Nevertheless, eating is still just as basic to our survival, each and every one of us, as to prehistoric societies, so we live with a kind of tension of non-recognition and non-appreciation that can be quite bizarre. Thus eating has become increasingly separated from survival and maintenance of life in our consciousness. For the most part, we eat with great automaticity and little insight into its critical importance for us in sustaining life, and also in sustaining health. We are driven far more by DESIRE than by NEED, our relationships to food shaped by social pressures, the advertising industry, agribusiness, food processing, and by conditioned taste preferences and portion sizes that, in first world countries and particularly the United States, have led to a virtual epidemic of obesity over little more than a decade.

Our eating is often driven by rather primordial urges and accompanied by equally primordial and extremely unconscious behaviors. Just think: we feed ourselves, and we have all had to learn to do it. And we do it all the time, not just to sustain our lives, but often out of sheer habit, and the urge to satisfy cravings that have little to do with real nourishment and often stem more from emotional discomfort than any actual hunger." (pp.230-3).

It's precisely this new relationship with food, placing our desire above our need that has resulted in our imbalanced relationship to food in modern, western society. Mindfulness aims to help redress the balance and re-establish equilibrium. I will now outline what I believe are the five major roadblocks to mindful eating. Most of us engage in these roadblocks on a daily basis without even being aware.

For each one, I will give you helpful tools you can use to bring more awareness to food and your experience of eating, an awareness that will help you to consistently overcome these roadblocks.

Roadblock #1: Distracted Eating

I expect you know what I'm talking about here. Who among us doesn't multitask on a daily basis and especially while we are eating? I have noticed that in our North American culture, the preparation and consuming of food seems to be little more than an inconvenience in our stressed-out, busy lives. I, myself, have become particularly adept at eating while driving, a habit, which not only takes the joy out of a meal but is dangerous. I liken it to talking on a cell phone while driving – a very bad habit, indeed.

Have you ever eaten while also doing any of the following?

- Watching television?

- Driving?

- Working at your job?

- Having an argument?

- Sitting at the computer?

- Walking?

- Talking on the phone?

You are not alone! Here are some statistics:

- North American adults spend an average of 1 hour and 12 minutes per day eating, yet they spend between 2 ½-3 hours per day watching television.

- 66% of Americans report regularly eating dinner in front of the television.

In his recent book, *In Defense of Food*, Michael Pollan links our habit of absent-minded eating to a new nutritional philosophy in what he calls "the age of nutritionism". According to Pollan, "the sheer abundance of food in America has fostered a culture of careless, perfunctory eating" which takes the pleasure out of eating. [3]

So, why should you eat mindfully?

You will eat less and get out of the habit of overeating

Americans have been gaining weight for quite some time. The most recent National Center for Health Statistics report found that 32% of all U.S. adults are obese according to the government's Body Mass Index (BMI) classification system. By contrast, just 23% of adults were classified as obese in government surveys taken from 1988 through 1994. Government surveys also find that the increase in weight is in part related to an increase in calorie and dietary intake. In short, *people are eating more.*[4]

If the mind is focused on more than one task while eating, the brain may not receive critical signs that regulate food intake. If the brain fails to receive important messages such as the sensation of taste and satisfaction, it may not register the event as "eating". When this happens, your brain continues to send out hunger signals, increasing your risk of overeating.

You will drastically improve your digestive health

Recent research has found that when our mind is distracted during a meal, the digestive process may be 30-40% less effective.[5]

3   Pollan, Michael. *In Defense of Food: An Eater's Manifesto.* New York: The Penguin Press, 2008.
4   Refer the Pew Research Center Publications website: <http://pewresearch.org/pubs/309/eating-more-enjoying-less>.
5   David, Marc. *The Slow Down Diet: Eating for Pleasure, Energy, and Weight Loss.* Rochester: Healing Arts Press, 2005.

Distracted Eating

Write a list of all the ways you distract yourself while eating.

For homework, I want you to practice eating without distraction.

To help you achieve this, here are my "top 10" strategies for mindful eating:

TOP 10 Strategies for Mindful Eating

1. Only eat while sitting.

2. Set a place for yourself at the table with a placemat, cutlery, napkin and a glass for a beverage.

3. When at work, eat away from your work area – i.e. in a lunchroom, restaurant or outside.

4. Eat with chopsticks – it will automatically slow you down.

5. Take a few deep breaths before you eat to calm and center yourself.

6. Chew each bite at least 30 times before swallowing.

7. Give thanks for your meal and appreciate that you have food to eat.

8. If you are eating with others, avoid upsetting conversation over meals and, instead, practice eating quietly and mindfully with the other person.

9. Turn off the phone at all mealtimes so you won't be interrupted.

10. Eat at the same time every day for each of your three meals and make sure it takes you a minimum of 20 minutes to eat a meal.

Roadblock #2: Eating Without Enjoyment

This is a topic that is dear to my heart. You see my mother, Marion Kane, is a food writer. In fact, she was the food editor of two major Canadian newspapers for a total of 17 years. So while most kids spent their evenings playing outside, I was busy dining in the finest restaurants of Toronto ordering lots of dishes to help my mum in her tasting ceremony which would either make said restaurant into the latest "hot spot" or else put it out of business in a matter of weeks. What delicious power!

Unlike me, my mother doesn't appear to struggle with what to eat, how much to eat or knowing when she's full. But still, I have managed to learn some important things from her when it comes to eating joyfully. In my mother's house, eating is a celebration: a time set aside to painstakingly prepare and enjoy a good meal.

In my mother's words:

> *We all have to eat. Most people prepare some of their own meals. Many of us are passionate about food and cooking. All of which explains why I love being a food writer: It so easily connects me with individuals of every age, colour, social status, shape and size. I've written about where and what Toronto taxi drivers like to eat – a story that led me to burger joints, an African take-out, South Asian eateries and a Jewish deli. I once checked our city's cops' top spots to nosh and, for another article, visited favourite haunts of local truckers. In a different vein, I talked to chefs who man high-end*

kitchens atop downtown skyscrapers for CEOs, and penned a feature about those who prepare the fare at local spas and health clubs. Food is the great equalizer and, from my experience, there's no better way to lift one's spirits or create a bond than sharing it with others.

Julia Child seemed to agree with my mother when she said,

Dining with one's friends and beloved family is certainly one of life's primal and most innocent delights, one that is both soul-satisfying and eternal.

A recent survey showed that Americans are eating more but enjoying it less. Just 39% of adults in this survey say they enjoy eating "a great deal", down from the 48% who said the same in a survey in 1989. Also, the survey found that the decline in enjoyment of eating has been greater among those who consider themselves "overweight" than among those who consider themselves "just about the right weight".[6]

In other words, when you're not happy with your body, you're not enjoying one of life's greatest pleasures – eating.

6   Refer the Pew Research Center Publications website: <http://pewresearch.org/pubs/309/eating-more-enjoying-less>.

Eating With Enjoyment

Describe an ideal eating experience. Describe in detail the atmosphere, table setting, location, type of food you'd be enjoying and whether you would be alone or with others.

Think about how you eat your meals now. Now, write down some things that you can do to make your day-to-day eating experiences more enjoyable.

Roadblock #3: Eating Things You Don't Want

How often have you had the experience of pigging out on something and, once you'd consumed most or all of it, realized you didn't even like it? I know I have. Eating things we don't really want is part of the "mindless eating" phenomenon that is so prevalent in our society.

We can easily fall into this trap when we're not paying attention to what and how we are eating. It's a common phenomenon; one that I recently heard someone refer to as a "snackcident".

Many of us learned as children that it was a sin to not eat everything on our plates, and some were even forced to eat everything they were given before being given permission to leave the table! But if you can go back in time and recapture some of your childhood eating memories, can you remember how repulsed you felt by certain foods? Mine was turnip. Just smelling cooked turnip was enough to make me run for cover when I was little.

As adults, and especially as dieters, we may have become increasingly disconnected with our true food likes and dislikes and will often eat things just because we think they are "good for us".

I'd like to help you reconnect with your inner child so that she can help you re-learn what foods "call to you" and those you'd rather avoid.

Eating Things I Don't Want

Make a list of foods you want but do not allow yourself to buy or eat.

What foods are you eating that you don't really want?

If you allowed yourself to have the foods you want, whenever you craved them, what do you think would happen?

For homework this week, I'd like you to try the following:

Buy one of the foods you want but don't allow yourself to have and eat it. Write about how you felt after eating it.

Avoid eating one thing you don't want to eat this week. Write about how you felt after choosing not to eat it.

Roadblock #4: Eating When You're Not Hungry

I'm guessing that this roadblock frequently trips you up.

I believe that so many of us eat when we're not hungry because we are no longer tuned into our basic physiology, our body and its needs.

Unlike many animals, we eat for many other reasons besides our body's signaling to us that it needs fuel. Sometimes we eat simply because the food is there. It's there so why not eat it?

How many parties have you gone to where you weren't hungry but ate stuff on the buffet table just because it looked good or simply because it was there and eating it seemed the thing to do?

I'd like to introduce you to a tool that I often use in my therapy practice with women who are trying to tune into their bodies' natural hunger cues. It's called the Hunger/Satiety Scale. [7]

Here's how it works

Hunger has a wide range of intensities. Pay attention to your hunger and fullness cues. Imagine hunger as a scale from 1 to 10 where 1 is hunger to the point of light-headedness, 5 is no hunger and 10 is "absolutely stuffed" to the point where you may even start to feel pain. Ideally, you want to stay in the middle of this range between slightly hungry and comfortably full. If you allow yourself to get too hungry, everything starts to look good and it's easy to overeat. On the other hand, if you are always eating before you feel hungry, you are ignoring the natural signals that help you maintain a regular body weight. It is important to stop eating *just before* you feel full because it

---

7   Adapted from the following website: <http://efed.aces.uiuc.edu/101/healthyeat.
html#hunger>.

takes time for the brain to get the fullness message. Some days you will be more active and require more energy than others, so respond to hunger cues appropriately.

Eating When I'm Not Hungry

Think back to the meals you ate today. Now, rate your hunger both before and after each meal and snack on a scale of 1 to 10.

Think back to the last time you had a food craving when you weren't hungry (you probably won't have to go back too far).

Now, write why you went for that particular food at that particular time.

Now, I want you to tune into the way in which you are currently eating. How often are you eating beyond satisfaction? How often do you stop eating before being completely satiated (i.e. full to excess)?

Here's a Homework Exercise:

To learn about satisfaction, at your next meal, try eating half
the food on your plate and then give yourself a rating of where
you are on the hunger/satiety scale.

If you are at number five or above, stop eating.

And, finally, Roadblock #5: Sneaking Food

This is a very important area to address, as there is a huge correlation to sneak-eating and problematic relationships with food and body image. In the 10+ years that I've been working as a therapist specializing in disordered eating, I have not yet met one client who has made peace with food and their body without stopping the "sneak-eating" habit.

Sneaking Food
Write a list of the ways in which you eat less than what you want because you are in the presence of others.

Write a list of the ways in which you currently sneak food.

Write a list of the specific foods you sneak. Is there an identifiable pattern to your sneaking (i.e. type of food, time of day, etc.)?

If so, identify/describe the pattern.

Write a list of the ways in which you hide your eating.

Is there a pattern? If so, identify/describe the pattern.

Some more Homework:

Commit to not sneaking food at least once this week and, instead, to eat it in full view of others. Then write about the experience here.

Describe what was it like to be truthful about what you eat.

5

the food-mood connection

I don't know about you but, for me, what I choose to eat and how I'm feeling are inextricably linked. When I'm feeling blue, nothing but macaroni and cheese will do. When I'm feeling angry, I want something hard and crunchy that makes a lot of noise like potato chips or rice cakes. When I'm feeling anxious, I often have an unsettled stomach and usually go for something light and creamy like a smoothie. When I'm ecstatically happy for some reason, I can either eat a lot or very little and food choices range from chocolate cake to a plain salad. PMS is in another category all by itself: when held hostage by my hormones, I can somehow plough my way through an entire bag of cheese puffs or a tub of ice cream.

For most women I know, how they feel about food is anything but neutral. How they see food, experience it and desire it can change, without warning, instantaneously. Our emotional state and what we eat are almost always linked and often unconsciously. We learn to soothe ourselves emotionally with food at a very young age; sometimes before we can even talk. Relatives often reward or punish us with food and, as little children, we learn that good behaviour means getting an edible treat; and, if we're bad, we're punished by not getting the food we really want.

As adults, we often mirror these early patterns with food and mood and the result is that we end up eating for emotional reasons rather than because we are truly hungry. We become confused about why we eat what we do, when we do, and often feel out of control when it comes to food and our eating habits.

In this chapter, I'd like to lead you through an exploration of how food and mood are connected in your own life and how this pattern began. Also, I'd like to look at certain emotions that women with food and body image issues often have trouble expressing and, then, provide you with the tools you need to become emotionally unstuck so that you'll no longer have to turn to eating as a way to cope with difficult feelings. Lastly, I'd like to give you some tips and strategies to nurture yourself emotionally without turning to food as a primary self-soothing strategy.

I'd like to begin our journey by putting the spotlight on what we learned about food and eating from our families of origin. I have yet to meet a woman struggling with food and body image who doesn't also come from a family that struggles with these same issues and, as a result, reinforces these issues among family members from generation to generation.

In my work, I have found that disordered eating is handed down by what family systems therapists call the "generational transmission process". A good starting point for healing our relationship with food is to become aware of those habits and tendencies we picked up from our families while growing up.

Let me share with you a little bit about my own struggles with food, body image and family to illustrate my point about the causative relationship between families of origin and eating disorders.

My struggles with food and the battle to accept my body's natural size and shape have been nothing less than an obsession throughout most of my life. Raised in a Jewish family where food and being slender were a major focus, I was put on my first diet at the tender age of eight. It seemed that most of my elders were consumed with what they ate (or didn't eat) and were vigilant about maintaining what was, in their view, an acceptable body size.

This was very confusing because, in my culture, food was at the center of every holiday, ritual and family gathering. Foods were even divided into "good" and "bad" categories and some were given almost godly status. In general, Jews love to cook, eat and celebrate around the dinner table and, in my family, this is how it was and still is. Food in Jewish culture equals love; to refuse something edible that a relative has made with great love is simply unacceptable. The two very loud, very clear but conflicting messages repeated to me frequently and with force while growing up were: "Eat more!" and "Eat less!" Little wonder my relationship with food was both confused and conflicted. As a result of these mixed messages, I developed a love/hate relationship to both food and my body.

Now, I'd like to guide you to a better understanding of the messages about food that you absorbed as a child and how these helped to shape your present relationship to food and your body.

Conjure up in your mind a memory of what meals were like in your family when you were growing up.

What was the family table like?

Who was normally present at the table when you ate the main meal of the day?

Draw the table and everyone that was there.

Who prepared the food? Who served the food?

Now, recall what the atmosphere was like around the family table at mealtime – was it pleasant, unpleasant, mixed?

Did you talk? Did others talk?

What manner of conversation took place at the family table during mealtime?

Did you normally eat everything on your plate? Were there any rules about wasting food?

Did you have a choice about what or how much you ate?

Was food used as a reward or punishment?

Do you remember any meals, in particular (holiday meals, for example)?

What was happening in the family at those times? Describe these in detail.

Was anyone in your family on a diet or obsessed with food and weight or how they looked?

If so, who was it?

What did you learn about food and your body from that person?

For the rest of the exercises in this chapter, I want you to get accustomed to using a very helpful tool for identifying emotional eating patterns and learning to change them by replacing them with healthier alternatives. I call this tool an *emotional eating diary*.

By using the emotional eating diary, consistently and regularly, you will begin to identify patterns and triggers that lead to emotional eating. This will give you the gift of awareness, awareness of your emotional state and its connection to your eating. This awareness is the key to achieving long-term, sustained change in your eating habits since, only once you're aware of something, can you then choose to change it.

emotional eating diary

Date & Time	
Degree of Hunger	
Food Eaten & How Much	
Where I Was at the Time	
What Just Happened	
What I did After Eating	
What I Was Feeling at the Time	
What I Really Needed Instead of Food	
How I Could Nurture Myself Without Food Next Time	

Now, I'd like to shift our attention to the emotions we so often stuff down with food as a result of emotional eating patterns acquired at an early age. Following are the three major emotions that women most frequently find themselves stuffing down.

Emotion #1: Anger

We, as women, are socialized as young girls to be considerate and nice at all costs and are discouraged from expressing anger or resentment. If we do express anger directly, we are frequently called "bitches", a label that many of us desperately try to avoid.

Often, when angry, we have a tendency to eat instead of focusing on what is "eating us". We suppress our anger because we've been taught that it's not feminine to express it. We stuff our anger down with food in an effort to cope with our unresolved feelings but, sadly, this doesn't rid us of our anger; it simply buries it. And, for as long as we refuse to deal with rather than repress our anger, for as long as we continue to prevent the natural, normal expression of anger, it will keep rearing its ugly little head. In the process, we will have done untold damage to our bodies – not to mention our psyches – by overeating. And now, our anger has our feelings of guilt and shame to keep it company.

Think back to the most recent time you ate out of anger. Using the emotional eating diary on the following page, and anger as the emotion you were feeling at the time, write answers to each question for each of the remaining rows.

emotional eating diary—angry eating

Date & Time	
Degree of Hunger	
Food Eaten & How Much	
Where I Was at the Time	
What Just Happened	
What I did After Eating	
What I Was Feeling at the Time	
What I Really Needed Instead of Food	
How I Could Nurture Myself Without Food Next Time	

A way to get out of the angry eating trap is to delay stuffing our faces with food. Even ten minutes delay will do. Instead of eating, simply sit down, take a deep breath and tune into what you're really feeling and what you need to do to let go of your anger. For this, I recommend using the emotional eating diary on a regular basis.

Another key to dealing with anger is to set boundaries. I have found, over the years, that women who struggle with food and body image often have a very hard time setting limits with others. Once we learn how to enforce boundaries and to practice setting them, consistently and regularly, our eating issues often improve dramatically.

Note: All of the following information on boundaries is from handouts I've acquired as a therapist over the years and unfortunately, I do not know the original sources from which they come. I do apologise for not referencing them properly.

I like this simple definition of boundaries: "Where you end and I begin".

Boundaries are limits that we can set with other people to let them know:

"This is how far I am willing to go."

"This is what I will or won't do for you."

"This is what I will not tolerate from you."

Let's say you have a friend who wants you to look after her kids more than you would like. Perhaps you don't mind doing it occasionally, but not every week. You could set a boundary with her by saying: "I really enjoy looking after your kids occasionally, but I have a very full schedule and can only do it once a month maximum". This is letting her know what you will and won't do for her and how far you are willing to go. Learning to set clear limits and staying within those limits consistently can significantly reduce your anger quotient.

Here are 10 Signs of Unhealthy Boundaries

1. Talking at an intimate level at the first meeting.

2. Falling in love with a new acquaintance.

3. Going against personal values or rights to please others.

4. Touching a person without asking.

5. Allowing someone to take as much as they can from you.

6. Letting others direct your life.

7. Falling apart so someone will take care of you.

8. Accepting food, gifts, touch or sex that you don't want.

9. Being overwhelmed by a person or preoccupied with thoughts of them.

10. Letting others describe your reality and/or define who you are.

Three Tips for Setting Boundaries with Others

1. When you identify that you need to set a limit with someone, do it clearly, preferably without anger and in as few words as possible. Offer a brief explanation if it makes sense to do so but avoid justifying, rationalizing or apologizing.

2. You will probably feel ashamed and afraid when you set boundaries. Do it anyway. People may not know that they are trespassing on your emotional territory. Also, people don't respect others whom they can use. People use those they can use and respect those they cannot use. Healthy limits benefit everyone. Children and adults will feel more comfortable around you if you have clear, explicit boundaries.

3. You'll be tested when you set boundaries. Plan on it. It doesn't do any good to set a boundary until you're ready to enforce it. Often, the key to boundaries isn't convincing other people you have limits – it's convincing yourself! Once you really know what your limits are, it won't be difficult to convince others. In fact, people often sense when you've reached your limit. You'll stop attracting so many boundary invaders. Keep in mind that things will change only when you decide to change.

   When we feel angry and complain a lot about something, this may be a clue telling us that we need to set some boundaries. The things we can't stand, don't like and even hate may be areas crying out for boundaries. These strong feelings are indicators of problems, like a flashing red light on the car dashboard.

We may also need to break through shame and fear to take care of ourselves. Other clues that we may need to set a boundary are feeling threatened, "suffocated" or victimized by someone. We may need to get angry to set a boundary, but we don't need to stay resentful to enforce it.

On the pages following, you'll find a writing exercise to help you with boundaries.

Pick something that you're constantly angry about or feel strongly about to the point where you want to rip someone's head off. (Hint: It will probably have to do with another person's behaviour.)

Write down whom it is that makes you feel this way and describe the behaviour that drives you crazy.

Now, write down why you haven't set a boundary with that person.

What are you afraid of or avoiding?

Now, write down a boundary that you could set around that behaviour and the person involved that would prevent you from feeling angry or resentful or victimized in the future.

Your homework is to enforce this boundary for the next week, regardless of how much you're tested, how guilty or ashamed you feel and how much it takes out of you.

Trust me it'll be worth it!

You'll know you've succeeded in setting your boundary when you no longer feel angry or resentful or victimized by the person engaging in the behaviour you can't stand. This person may continue behaving that way forever, but it won't matter to you because you'll have a boundary in place to protect yourself from it.

Emotion #2: Anxiety

Have you ever eaten because you were scared, nervous or generally restless?

You are not alone. Many of us eat in an attempt to lower anxiety. It's a coping mechanism, a way of self-medicating ourselves. In fact, recent research has shown that carbohydrate rich foods like bread and cookies actually boost serotonin – a chemical that makes you feel calm – levels in the brain. This explains why we often reach for carbohydrate rich or "comfort foods" when we're stressed.

Unfortunately, this calming effect only lasts for a brief time. Soon after we've eaten, the serotonin levels begin to fall and the anxiety comes back in full-force. Then we're not only left with the original anxiety, but also the self-loathing and physical discomfort that accompany emotional eating.

Here are three things you can do instead of running to the refrigerator the next time you feel stressed and out of sorts:

Have a nap or go to bed early
Research has shown that people who are well rested are less susceptible to anxiety and stress and are better at resisting the urge to overeat. For some reason, not sleeping enough messes with our internal temperature regulating mechanism and putting food into our system brings it back into balance. Therefore, being tired can trigger the urge to overeat.

Make sure you get at least 8 ½ hours of sleep each night to reduce the urge to overeat in your waking hours.[1]

---

1   Webb, D. "What's Eating You? The Five Reasons We Reach for Food (When We're Not Hungry) and How to Stop It". New Woman March 1998, 50-52.

Do something relaxing and calming

We all have different ways of relaxing. Some people like to paint. Others like to go for a long walk or sit in silence and breathe deeply. In the next chapter, I will be covering this aspect of finding peace with food and our bodies in depth. But, for now, I'd like you to write down at least five activities that help you feel relaxed and calm.

1.

2.

3.

4.

5.

The next time you feel stressed and anxious and instinctively turn to food, resist the urge to run to the cupboard or fridge and, instead, practice one of the relaxing activities you have identified on this list.

Fill out an emotional eating diary entry in order to figure out what's causing your anxiety in the first place. If you do this frequently enough, you'll start to notice patterns in your mood-food connections and can then identify specific triggers that make you susceptible to turning to food when you're stressed.

Once you know what those triggers are, you can come up with some concrete strategies to decrease your stress levels without resorting to placating yourself with food. You will soon learn that it's not food that you need in times of stress and anxiety, but something deeper and more satisfying – such as relaxation and stillness.

Think back to the most recent time you ate out of anxiety. Using the emotional eating diary below and anxiety as the emotion you were feeling at the time, write answers to each of the questions in each of the remaining rows.

emotional eating diary—anxious eating

Date & Time	
Degree of Hunger	
Food Eaten & How Much	
Where I Was at the Time	
What Just Happened	
What I did After Eating	
What I Was Feeling at the Time	
What I Really Needed Instead of Food	
How I Could Nurture Myself Without Food Next Time	

Emotion #3: Sadness

Even people who don't have major food issues sometimes overeat when they are feeling blue, the major difference being that it happens once in a blue moon not every time they feel bummed out. Within certain limits, it's a perfectly normal human urge.

But for those of you who eat when you're feeling sad on a regular basis, it can become a vicious cycle: you eat because you're depressed, then you feel even more depressed because you've eaten so much and your self-esteem plummets to an all-time low which can lead to a "what the hell" attitude increasing the likelihood of overeating when the next bout of the blues hits. Before you know it, you're caught in a hellish self-perpetuating cycle and it can be very difficult to get out of it once it's started.

Here are some ways to deal with 'the blues' that will make you feel a whole lot better than eating:

Talk it out

If you're feeling blue, it probably has something to do with an upsetting incident that has happened and you may feel a whole lot better to get it off your chest by calling up a friend and sharing what you're feeling. Even if they can't do anything to make the situation better, just providing a listening ear, support and some encouragement can make you feel more positive about whatever it is that is bothering you.

According to a recent survey conducted by the British Mental Health Foundation, the most common way to beat a bad day is having someone to talk to. The survey found talking to another person was the top choice to lift the spirits, with 75% of people

(83% of women, 68% of men) choosing this as the best way to feeling better.[2]

Exercise

Research has shown, over and over again, that one of the best ways to battle the blues is by simply moving your body and getting your heart pumping. Even doing just 30 minutes of moderate exercise boosts the feel-good chemicals in the brain. Physical activity actually alters our brain chemistry and can leave you feeling a whole lot lighter and brighter emotionally.

Some research studies indicate that regular exercise may be as effective as other treatments like medication to relieve mild to moderate depression. This is because exercise boosts the production of serotonin, an important brain chemical (neurotransmitter) that contributes to a range of functions, including sleep and wake cycles, libido, appetite and mood. Some researchers have found that regular exercise, and the increase in physical fitness that results, alters serotonin levels in the brain and leads to improved mood and feelings of well-being.[3]

"Boo Hoo" It Out

This is the non-technical term for having a "pity party for one". Really indulge yourself here. I like to run a hot bath with lots of bubbles and light candles. I put Billie Holiday on the stereo singing pathetic songs about lost love, discrimination and life's general unfairness. I sob myself silly. Before long, I'm smiling again. Then, I start to laugh and, before long, I find myself feeling a whole lot lighter and more optimistic. Surprisingly (or

---

2   Refer: <http://www.truestarhealth.com/members/cm_archives03ML4P1A98. html

3   Refer: <http://www.betterhealth.vic.gov.au/bhcv2/bhcarticles.nsf/pages/Depression_and_exercise?OpenDocument>.

not surprisingly), flannel pajamas and fuzzy slippers can also do wonders for "sadness of the soul".

The belief that crying has positive effects is of ancient origin. More than two thousand years ago, Aristotle theorized that crying at a drama cleanses the mind of suppressed emotions by a process called catharsis, the reduction of distress by releasing the emotions. Many people attend movies and plays that they know beforehand are tearjerkers. Such people may cry freely in movies and may delight in the experience for the emotional release it offers.

The human body actually makes three different kinds of tears: basal tears for simple eyeball lubrication, reflex tears to wash away irritants (onion fumes, debris specks or hits to the eye), and emotional tears. Weeping tears contain various hormones that the other tears don't and 20% to 25% more protein.

Scientists don't yet know why emotional tears differ but it's interesting that they do. Some hypothesize that these tears may wash the body clean of wastes.

Think back to the most recent time you ate out of sadness. Now, using the emotional eating diary on the following page, and sadness as the emotion you were feeling at the time, write answers for each heading in each of the remaining rows.[4]

---

4   Refer: <http://www.physicsforums.com/showthread.php?t=39324>>.

emotional eating diary—sad eating

Date & Time	
Degree of Hunger	
Food Eaten & How Much	
Where I Was at the Time	
What Just Happened	
What I did After Eating	
What I Was Feeling at the Time	
What I Really Needed Instead of Food	
How I Could Nurture Myself Without Food Next Time	

Before we go any further, I would like to cover some other issues that lead to emotional eating:

Let's start with that fussy little demon, *perfectionism*.

I have yet to meet a woman who struggles with food and body image who isn't, to some extent or another, a perfectionist. I have found, in all my years of therapy work, no exceptions to this rule.

Maybe, someday, I'll be proven wrong but, until then, I will continue giving women tools to overcome perfectionism in order to find peace with food and their bodies.

Perfectionism can best be defined as "an attitude or set of beliefs that involve setting unrealistic and unattainable goals".

Perfectionist thinking usually involves "should thinking" like: "I should be thinner." or "I should be the perfect wife/mother/daughter/whatever." or "I should be able to eat like a normal person." [5]

Do you "should on yourself" constantly?

I thought you might.

Following is a useful writing exercise to help you with your "shoulding" problem.

---

5   *McNamara, Kathleen, *Improving Eating Behaviour and Body Image: A Structured Group Program for Repeat Dieters and Others at Risk for an Eating Disorder*. Department of Psychology Colorado State University, 1986.

Write a list of your favourite "I should" statements. Call it "My Favourite Shoulds".

Now, take a look at your list. How many of your "shoulds" are realistic and attainable? How many just plain ridiculous?

On this page, I want you to take each of your favourite "shoulds" and turn it into a realistic and attainable goal.

It helps to set specific rather than general goals and to omit the "shoulds" in your should statements. Change "should" to "will".

For example, where you might have written something like: "I should be the perfect mother."

Change it to read:

"In the next two weeks, I will set aside two hours a week to spend with my child(ren). "

Do this with each of your "shoulds" and see how your "should" list has been transformed into a list of very realistic and attainable goals.

This brings us to a concept I'd like to share with you that can be particularly helpful in overcoming perfectionism. It's called: *lowering our standards* .

Recovery, Inc. is an international self-help group that assists people in overcoming anxiety disorders. Here is a Recovery saying that I really love:

"Lower your standards and your performance will rise."

Simply put, the less we try to be perfect and just strive to do a good enough job of something, the better we end up doing.

This is exemplified nicely in the book, *Too Perfect: When Being in Control Gets Out of Control.* In it, the authors encourage readers to let go of trying to be an "A+" and lower their expectations of themselves to a "B" instead.

When I suggest doing this to my perfectionist clients, they often gasp and say, "That's impossible!" My answer to that is, "No it's not. It's just challenging. What really is impossible is living up to the unrealistic expectations you set for yourself."

On the following pages you'll find some written exercises to help you get from an A+ to B and feel good about it.

In what areas of your life could you lower you standards a little bit? Make a list.

If you were to just do a good enough job in these areas, how would it make you feel?

What difference would it make in your life?

What about your life would change for the better?

Who would benefit from these changes and how?

Who would benefit from these changes and how?

homework

For your homework, pick one area that you identified as need-
ing a lowering of standards and practice being a "B" instead of
an "A+" in that area this week.

Then, write about what it was like and the benefits you received as a result of this lowering of standards in the space
below.

Let's look now at a phenomenon plaguing so many of us, something I like to call *fearing our power*.

I break it down into two basic categories:

1. Fear of Being "Too Much"

2. Fear of Taking Up Space.

These two categories or fears often go hand-in-hand. Find one and you probably don't have far to look to find the other.

Here is a fabulous excerpt called "Fear of Being Too Much" from the book *Succulent Wild Woman*, by SARK:

> *All my life, I've heard that I'm 'too much'. Too wild, too loud, too outrageous, too emotional, too sensitive, too needy, TOO MUCH. As I age, I see the temptation to laugh a bit less loudly, ask less, and tone it down for the benefit of others. Often I don't even know who these others are but they might be upset, so I comply.*
>
> *I was actually warned in a restaurant one time for laughing too loudly! The manager came over and said crabbily, 'Some of my customers are annoyed by your laughter – why don't you keep it down?' I asked who these customers were. He refused to say, so I stood up and said, 'Could I see a show of hands of people that are upset by the sound of my laughter?' No one raised their hands, so I said to the manager, 'Good. The matter is settled.'[6]*

6   SARK, Succulent Wild Women. (New York: Fireside, 1997) 46-7.

So let's risk being guilty of wearing something that's a bit "too much", of laughing "too much" and of loving "too much".

Written Exercises: "Being Too Much"
Close your eyes for a moment and go back in your mind and pick out a memory of a time when you feared being "too much". Write about this memory in detail.

In the end, did you take the risk of being "too much"? Do you have any regrets?

If you didn't take the risk, write about the consequences you suffered as a result.

If you did take the risk, write about what you gained from the experience.

homework

For your homework, make a list of all the ways you can practice being "too much" in your journal and actually do one of
them this week.

Now I'd like to explain the second fear category: "Fear of Taking Up Space". I believe there is a direct link between body size and personal power in our society. And I do not think it a mere coincidence that, physically, women are expected to take up as little room as is humanly possible.

I can't tell you how many times clients struggling with anorexia tell me that they don't want to "take up space" but want to "be small" or "disappear." The alarming metaphors that many women use in this regard point to the fact that women are somehow conditioned to think that they need to shrink physically in order to be accepted as members in good standing of the human species.

Here's a quote from Susan Brownmiller's book, *Femininity*, that illustrates the push-pull we do as women with what we are expected to be versus what we actually are physically:

> *Fleshiness, as we know, is problematic to the present-day feminine illusion, for while fat creates the celebrated dimorphic curves of womanhood, it is also the agent of massiveness and bulk, properties more readily associated with masculine solidity and power. What seems to be a natural tendency of the female body to acquire substantial, if wobbly, mass runs counter to the preferred ideal of delicate shapeliness.*[7]

I'm not going to enter into a detailed discussion of where this whole concept came from, as we'll be covering that at length in the chapter about body image. But, for the purposes of this chapter and your own healing, I think it's important to start making the connection between size and personal power so that you can begin right away to start questioning the valid-

---

7   Brownmiller, S. *Femininity*. (London: Paladin, 1984) 16-17.

ity of society's "thinness imperative" and start challenging it by fighting back.

Who came up with a "size zero" anyway? That's a relatively new concept, I believe. What message are we sending to women and girls when we idealize the fantasy of being a size zero? In my view, we're literally telling them that they need to be nothing, to disappear.

A message like that certainly doesn't encourage women to want to stand up tall with head held high and take on the world now, does it?

Written Exercises: "Fear of Taking up Space"

Identify the ways in which you endeavor to make yourself "small" and, as best you can, list the reasons you do it.

What are some ways you can begin to take up more space in the world and in your life?

How will you know when you are no longer "playing small" in life?

What will your life look like then?

What will have changed?

Describe the person you will have become.

Nurturing Myself Without Food

I'd like to end this chapter by exploring how we can begin nurturing ourselves without food. In other words, how we can meet our emotional needs without stuffing our feelings down with food.

Make a list of the things you could do to nurture yourself when you feel like reaching for food for emotional reasons.

Here are some suggestions for nurturing yourself without food gathered from my clients over the years:

Ways to nurture yourself without food

- Take a hot bubble bath surrounded by candles

- Curl up with a teddy bear and cry until you can't cry anymore

- Watch a sad or funny movie

- Pet and cuddle a cat or a dog

- Listen to lullabies and gently rock yourself to sleep

- Go for a long walk in nature

- Pray

- Meditate

- Do yoga

- Call a friend and ask them to listen

- Rip up old phonebooks to let out anger

- Turn on the stereo and dance around the living room

- Buy yourself a piece of clothing or jewelry

- Read a good book

- Write in your journal

- Get dressed up just for the hell of it

- Go swimming

- Colour

- Give yourself a foot massage with peppermint foot lotion

- Write a letter

- De-clutter and/or clean your home

- Decorate

- Punch a pillow

- Be lazy without feeling guilty

- Draw a picture

- Take photos

- Browse in stores you love

- Write positive affirmations about yourself

- Giggle until you have tears running down your cheeks

- Go to the park or beach

- Play with children

- Volunteer your time to help others

- People watch

- Buy yourself a bouquet of your favorite flowers

meditation & relaxation

In this chapter, we are going to explore Meditation and Relaxation in detail. We'll learn what they're all about and why they are particularly useful tools for women who struggle with food and body image. We'll also have a chance to experience several of these powerful techniques and practices first-hand.

In his groundbreaking book, *The Slow Down Diet: Eating for Pleasure, Energy, and Weight Loss*, author Marc David makes a direct connection between stress and weight gain. He explains what he calls the 'metabolic power of relaxation' when he states:

> *The same part of our brain that turns on stress turns off digestion. And conversely, the part of the brain that turns on the relaxation response turns on full, healthy digestive power. Eating healthy food is only half of the story of good nutrition. Being in the ideal state to digest and assimilate food is the other half.* [1]

1   David, Marc. *The Slow Down Diet: Eating for Pleasure, Energy and Weight Loss.* (Rochester: Healing Arts Press, 2005) 19.

In other words, you can eat all the lettuce and sprouts in the world but, if you're stressed out when you're eating them, you won't digest them properly and your body won't be able to utilize the nutrients they provide. On the other hand, if you eat a greasy burger and fries when you're calm and relaxed, you'll be able to digest and properly assimilate what nutrients there are to be found in a burger and fries. And here's something else from Marc David to think about the next time you think that going on a diet or restricting certain "fattening foods" is a good idea:

> *Worrying about fat increases fat. Anxiety about weight loss causes your body to put fat on and retain it. In medical terms, chronic stress decreases thermic efficiency – your ability to burn calories and metabolize stored fat. It is totally counterproductive to stress yourself out about weight loss because the same stress causes you to put weight on.*[2]

I can actually hear you thinking: "What? No way!"

When I read that, I was surprised myself. How could worry increase fat in the body? Well, apparently it does. The body is an amazing machine and we still know very little about the intricacies between the body and the mind. We're simply at the beginning of a new frontier of discoveries in this field and it's simply... well...mind-blowing.

So the long and the short of it is that the more you obsess about what foods you're eating and not eating, count calories mathematician-style and weigh yourself like a maniac, the more you're going to keep the weight. The less you worry about all that stuff and relax, the more weight you will lose.

---

2   Ibid, 28.

Do you ever wonder why the French eat such high-fat foods and stay at a reasonable weight? This may be a clue!

This brings me to why we're spending an entire chapter exploring meditation and relaxation.

You paid some of your hard-earned cash to purchase this book and to learn some tools to help you get the "food/weight monster" off your back and to find some peace amidst the craziness in this diet-obsessed world of ours. Well, here are two of the greatest tools I can offer you, themselves worth the price of admission in my opinion – meditation and relaxation.

From new scientific research, we now know that the more oxygen you breathe in the more fully you burn calories consumed in food.[3] Not only that, but you feel a whole lot calmer and more peaceful as a result. There's a reason that the ancient practices of yoga and meditation have been around for so long and are so popular – they work!

So why do we find it so hard to regularly incorporate practices into our daily life that bring us such bliss, relaxation and peace? Because we're great at making excuses, that's why! Have you ever defended yourself against doing yoga, meditating or having a short nap with any of the following arguments/excuses?

"I don't have the time. I have too much to do."

"I can't do that because it's selfish."

"It's not a priority, I'll do it tomorrow."

And on and on…

---

3   Ibid, 36.

Well, starting right now, none of those excuses are going to wash because, within the pages of this book you are being held captive; you are my prisoner and I'm going to make you try some of these restorative and life-changing practices whether you like it or not. As one of my yoga teachers often says – "No excuses! Just Do It!"

I don't know if you know this already but yoga was actually invented as a tool to prepare the body and mind for the highly disciplined practice of sitting meditation. By stretching and moving the body before we sit in stillness, we let go of tightness in the body and can even release pent-up feelings so that we are looser and more relaxed before sitting.

I want to talk with you now about yoga, the mind-body practice that I have been doing regularly for almost two decades. I discovered the magic of yoga when I was 19, in my first year of university. I was in the throes of a serious eating disorder and was looking for something to give me a sense of peace. After my first yoga class, I was hooked. I have yet to find another mind-body practice that leaves me feeling so good afterwards.

Throughout the years, I have tried every form of yoga imaginable in my quest for body/mind balance and have enjoyed most of them immensely. The one that I keep coming back to at least three times a week, however, is the most basic and simple form of yoga called "Hatha".

Throughout my journey as a devoted and eager yoga student, I have heard many definitions of what yoga is but the simplest one that speaks to me the most is that yoga is the union of mind and body and that, by practising yoga, we are given the tools we need to attain and maintain balance between our heads and our physical body. Hatha yoga attempts to balance mind and body via physical exercises or "asanas" involving controlled breathing and the calming of the mind through relaxation and meditation. [4]

In western society, I feel that we need this balance more than anyone else in the world. So many of us live in our heads, thinking ourselves silly. I have found that, as a therapist, one of the greatest gifts I can share with clients is the benefits of practicing ancient mind-body connection methods such as yoga. I urge all the women I counsel in my practice, no matter what their personal issue, to give yoga a try. After ten years, I have yet to get any negative feedback based on their experiences!

When it comes to issues around food and body image, yoga is a winner indeed.

A recent study found that mind-body exercise, and yoga in particular, is associated with greater body satisfaction and fewer symptoms of disordered eating than traditional aerobic exercise like jogging or using cardio machines. Yoga practitioners reported less self-objectification, greater satisfaction with physical appearance and fewer disordered eating attitudes compared to non-yoga practitioners.

Why is this? It's because during yoga, a woman learns to tune into her body and listen to how it is feeling and what it needs. This helps us to turn our gaze inward rather than focusing so much on how we look on the outside. When we focus more on our inner selves, we become less preoccupied by what we look like on the surface.

---

4   Refer: <http://en.wikipedia.org/wiki/Hatha_yoga>.

Also, through the practice of yoga, we come to respect and appreciate our bodies in a whole different way. The focus isn't so much on how our body looks but what it is capable of doing, feeling and experiencing. The study cited states that this leads to a more positive body image and healthier eating habits in women who practice yoga regularly. This was not the case for women who focused on aerobic exercise exclusively. They were much less satisfied with their bodies' appearance and struggled more with healthy eating habits.

What is so exciting about the results of this study is the finding that, through yoga, women may intuitively discover a way to buffer themselves against messages that tell them that having a thin and toned body leads to happiness and success.[5]

I am not, nor do I pretend to be, a certified yoga teacher so I will not present any yoga postures in this book. But I strongly suggest you try out some yoga and soon. Either take a class or two in your local community or choose from a wide array of videos, DVD's and CD's, which will guide you through an entire practice. For the purposes of what we're trying to achieve here, I suggest you try Hatha or Yin Yoga to begin with. These are, in my experience, the most basic and calming forms of yoga and have proven to be highly effective for women who want to find peace with food and their bodies.

In the rest of this chapter, I want to focus on two things only: prayer and meditation. Why? Firstly, because I believe it is these two things combined that saved me, personally, from death by eating disorder and so I naturally think them important and, secondly, because I have found confirmation in my

---

5   Daubenmier, Jennifer Joan. *A Comparison of Hatha Yoga and Aerobic Exercise on Women's Body Satisfaction.* Dissertation Abstracts International (Mar 2003, B 63/09) 4415.

work as a therapist over the years that prayer and meditation are invaluable tools that have the power to heal and transform lives in astounding ways.

For clarification's sake, I am saying all of this as a person who comes from a long line of scientists, medical doctors and academics. I was raised in a family where things had to be scientifically proven to have any credibility whatsoever. In short, I am not very susceptible to "New-Ageology" even in my most open-minded state. However, I have also had some terribly challenging things happen throughout my life and putting my faith in science did not lead to any comfort or peace during these tough times. Praying and meditating, however, did.

Through prayer and meditation, I discovered the key difference between "being in one's head" as opposed to "being in one's body". I'm guessing that many of you are like me and are more in your head than your body, trying to reason everything out, think things through and find solutions to all of life's problems with your cerebral cortex. Let me ask you a question: how's that working for you?

If being in your head worked for you, you wouldn't be reading this book trying to learn some new problem-solving tools! One thing that I've learned ever so painfully and without much grace is that having a good head on my shoulders has it's pluses, but being intelligent is oftentimes a curse when it comes to being happy and peaceful. No matter how hard I might try, I simply cannot reason or think myself into a peaceful or happy state!

In my own personal journey towards wholeness, one thing that has helped me more than anything else is the belief in a power greater than myself. Call it "God"; "the Creator", "Universal

Life Force" or whatever else speaks to you. All I know is that millions of people throughout the centuries and around the globe have put their faith in a higher power and it has done wonders for them.

This was not an easy step for me to take either. I come from a family of Jewish radicals, socialists and non-believers. They gave up on believing in something greater than themselves after being persecuted, murdered and segregated for hundreds of years and I can definitely see why. Their argument has significant merit – how could an all-powerful, all-loving God let six million of our people be murdered in the Holocaust?

I guess that one of the benefits of not having any religious upbringing whatsoever was having a spiritual clean slate, so to speak, to work with. So I decided that, while organized religion isn't for me, a spiritual connection is. I have been using prayer and meditation daily for almost two decades. What are the benefits I've enjoyed as a result? They are too numerous to list and many of them cannot even be put into words so I will resist trying. What I will say is that through daily prayer and meditation over the years, I have been able to let go of a life-threatening eating disorder permanently and have found a sense of peace, calm and tranquility that I never knew, or thought, possible. For me, there is no going back.

One of my greatest inspirations has been Marianne Williamson, another Jewish woman-centered spiritual seeker, who talks and writes with great enthusiasm about a work called, *A Course in Miracles*. I have tried to read the *Course* and study it on my own with little success, as I felt it was written in a foreign language. I feel that Marianne Williamson is a fabulous interpreter of this great work and makes it user-friendly by adding humour and personal anecdotes that everyone can relate to. I highly recommend that you read her books and listen to her audiotapes as well.

According to Ms. Williamson: "Prayer is when we talk to God and meditation is when we listen." So, for now, we'll start with talking to a power greater than ourselves and then move on to listening for the answers we are seeking.

In her book, *The Flowering of The Soul: A Book of Prayers By Women*, Lucinda Vardey defines prayer in this way:

> *Prayer is absolute, unmixed attention and focus on the Divine. It can be in the form of praise, yearning, pleading, seeking, supplication, or listening. It can be in thought, in words, in feelings, in emptiness, in surrender, in movement. Prayer is consciously and attentively giving and receiving love and grace. Prayer guides us to live actively by divine inspiration. Prayer is the anchor of connectedness with all that matters, and a means to eternal existence. Prayer reminds us of how small we are, and of how much help we need. Prayer is a force that lifts our hearts and infuses them with purity and openness. Prayer is the interior conversation that sustains us and promotes the 'flowering of the soul'.*

I suggest to clients that they make a time to sit and pray twice a day, once upon waking in the morning and once before going to bed at night. When you do this in the morning, you are making a positive and directed intention for how you want to handle whatever comes your way during the course of your waking hours. And when you sit down to pray and meditate after the day is done, you are putting closure on all that has happened during the day and infusing all the day's experiences with a positive and spiritual focus.

Unless you've been doing this for quite some time on a regular and consistent basis, I cannot possibly convey to you in words what powerful changes can take place as a result. And the time it takes each day? Twenty minutes – tops! That's one sitcom without all of the commercials! Now, who can honestly say they can't carve out 20 minutes a day to assure themselves of a calm mind and a peaceful attitude? The benefits are not only for ourselves but for those around us whom we love too.

So, to get you started, I want to share with you some of my favourite prayers that have given me a positive outlook and so much peace and healing over the years.

The first three prayers are by Marianne Williamson and come from her book, *Illuminata: Thoughts, Prayers, Rites of Passage*. This is one of the best books of prayer I have found and I suggest you pick up a copy of this amazing book for your own use.

Here is a morning prayer to start your day called, *A New Day*.

A New Day

Dear God,
Thank you for this new day, its beauty and its light.
Thank you for my chance to begin again.
Free me from the limitations of yesterday.
Today may I be reborn.
May I become more fully a reflection of your radiance.
Give me strength and compassion and courage and wisdom.
Show me the light in myself and others.
May I recognize the good that is available everywhere.
May I be, this day, an instrument of love and healing.
Lead me into gentle pastures.
Give me deep peace that I might serve you most deeply.
Amen.

Here is an evening prayer to end your day called, *Evening Prayer*."

Evening Prayer

Dear God,
I surrender to you the day now over.
May only the love remain.
Take all else into the fire of your transformative power.
Release me; release others, from any effects of my wrong-mindedness.
As I now give to you who I am, what I did,
Who I loved, whom I failed to love.
Please make all things right.
Take all things.
May I continue to grow in your light and love.
Tomorrow, may I be better.
Amen.

And here is a lovely prayer to remind you of who you are called, *Prayer for Myself.*

Prayer for Myself

Dearly beloved God,
In whom I lay my trust,
Please give me new life.
Fill every cell of my being, transform each
 thought, cleanse every heartbeat,
That I might be as you would have me be.
Take away the darkness of my past.
Fill me with your blessing and graciousness.
Allow me rebirth from the many deaths I have endured in this
life.

Dear God,
I have been through the wars.
Where I have been weak, please make me strong.
Where I perceive myself as guilty, please show
 me my wound and take from me its sting.
May I experience the beauty, the abundance, the
 power and the joy that is your wish for all mankind,
That I might be a vessel for these things in the lives of others.

The wicked in myself and others has tormented me.
Please cast away that darkness from my life.
I know yours is the power,
I know yours are the holy truths, the currents of love
 and power that remain,
And so I ask, dear God, please remove the burdens on my
heart,
Cast out the demons from my mind and my environs.
May I see the light at the center of my being.

I believe in your power within me.
I know it is there.

Dear God, help me find it.
I have faith in your light.
Please show it to me that I might give up the
 fight to be anything other than who I am.
May I fly with angels and sing with angels and
know the angels in myself and others

Henceforth and forever as you have promised.
Please hold my hand.
Please take me home.
Please move me forward.
Thank you.
Amen.

I wrote the following prayer for myself and all of the women
out there who struggle to accept the unique and sacred "package"
they happen to come in – their bodies.

A Prayer of Thanks for the Body

Oh Great Mother,
Creator,
Goddess of all,
Earth, Sea, Sky, and mountains,
I thank you for giving me this body.
It is my home,
My sanctuary,
The vehicle
In which I journey through life
Every day that I am alive.

Thank you for my eyes,
Which allow me to see the beauty all around me,
As well as the suffering
Which serves to open my heart that little bit more
So that I can extend compassion and love
All around me.

Thank you for my ears,
Those magical instruments which
Give me the ability to hear the voices around me,
Sweet music, birds singing, a cat's soothing purr,
And the sound of ocean waves lapping on the shore.

Thank you for my nose,
The miracle which allows me to smell a rose,
The salty ocean,
A delicious home-cooked meal…
Taking long, slow, rhythmic breaths,
In and out,
Letting go,
Further and further,
Into deep relaxation and stillness.

Thank you for my mouth,
Which gives me the power to speak my truth,
How I'm feeling,
What I'm thinking,
What I want and need.
To kiss and to be kissed,
Connecting me to those I love so much.

Thank you for my arms which
Allow me to hold another close,
To touch and caress,
And show them my love.

Thank you for my legs and feet
Which allow me to move gracefully
From one place to the next.
These legs and feet have taken me to so many amazing places
And will take me to so many more.

Thank you for all of my curves,
My breasts,
My belly,
My hips,
My buttocks,
For they remind me that I am a woman
Beautiful,
Sexy,
Sensual,
Strong,
Flowing,
Warm,
Soft,
And open.

Thank you for this body made in your image-
I, too, am a Goddess
Standing strong,
Proud,
Radiant,
All Loving,
All-powerful,
All knowing,

And full of life-giving magic.
Like you, I have been given
The awe-inspiring ability to create life,
In all its many forms.
My womb is a sacred space
Which feeds, nurtures
And gives birth to endless possibilities.

Thank you for making me a woman
And for reminding me of who I really am
Your daughter
A perfect,
Innocent,
Brilliant,
And blessed child of the Great Goddess.

Thank you mother for bringing me home to you.
Here, I am safe and protected in your arms.
Here, I know I am loved unconditionally.
Here, I can make mistakes and still be loved.
Here, I can truly shine and become the incredible
Woman you created me to be.
Amen.

Now, I'd like you to write your own prayer; one that speaks to you personally. Now that we've gone over some prayers together, you should have an idea of the basic format.

homework

Say your prayer at least once a day, either in the morning or the evening, for one week and then write in the space below what you experienced as a result.

In his book, *Mindfulness, Bliss, and Beyond*, Ajahn Brahm gives a description of meditation, which really speaks to me. He describes the meditative state as a "letting go of our burdens". He says that during meditation, you are given the opportunity to "unload as much baggage as you can" (p.2). When I hear this definition, my shoulders automatically drop a few centimeters at the relief promised!

Now, I'd like to give you a taste of this sweet feeling by providing you with a deep and restful and extremely rejuvenating meditation. I suggest that you record yourself reading the following meditation and then play it back to yourself when you want to drift away. You can also purchase a downloadable MP3 audio version of me reading this by going to: www.endyoureatingdisorder.com. You should lie down for this, either on a bed or couch or on a comfortable mat on the floor with a pillow supporting your head.

This is a time of complete relaxation. A conscious effort to relax as completely as possible. Get into as comfortable a position as you can and close your eyes. For the next couple of minutes, just concentrate on your breathing. Take deep, slow belly breaths – in through the nose and out through the nose. Start by filling your belly with air and then moving it up into your lungs, all the way through your throat and then out through your nose.

Be aware that there's no right or wrong way to do what you're doing now, whatever results you get are perfect results and, if all you do is relax, that's wonderful. This is not a time to be worrying about any of the things that are happen¬ing in your day-to-day life. This is a time only for you, where you can let everything else go. For this short period of time, you can completely relax. You are in complete control. You are completely safe and secure.

If, at any point, your mind drifts away just bring it slowly back to where you are. In your body. Right here. Right now. If you hear my voice, that's fine; and, if you don't, that's fine too. You can be absolutely sure that your subconscious is hearing every word I say.

And now, in your mind's eye, I'd like you to imagine a word all lit up in the night sky. That word is RELAX. Just relax...that's all you have to do – nowhere to go, nothing to do. Simply BEING. Right here. Right now.

Now, release the weight of your body onto the support of the floor.

Notice how your back makes contact with the support of the floor.

Relax the back of your legs...the back of your hips... your lower back, middle back, and upper back. Feel the weight and relaxation of the back of your body sinking into the floor.

Relax the back of your shoulders... the back of your arms...the back of your neck... and the back of your head. Wiggle and make any adjustments needed to relax the back of your body into the ground more fully. Melt into the support of the floor beneath you completely.

Now, notice the weight of your body. Notice the weight of your legs as they rest on the floor. Let your legs be heavy. Let your thighs, feet and toes relax. Release, relax and let go of them completely. Let your legs drift and float and now forget about them.

Notice the weight of your hips and pelvis, as they rest on the floor. Let the weight of your pelvis sink into the floor.

Notice the weight of your rib cage. Let the back ribs melt into the floor. Feel your abdomen expand with each inhalation. As you exhale, let the belly fully contract…like a giant balloon inflating and then completely deflating…relaxing deeper with each breath.

Notice the weight of your shoulders and arms as they rest on the floor. Let your arms be so heavy that they sink through the floor. Then release them completely. Let go. Let them drift and float away and then forget about them.

Notice the weight of your head, as it rests on the floor. Let the head be heavy. Feel your neck and throat release and relax.

Relax the muscles of your face…relax your eyes and eyelids …your cheeks melt into relaxation…release, relax, let go of your jaw …feel your forehead and eyebrows smooth and relax… feel your scalp melt into relaxation…your whole head and face totally relaxed, released.

You may be surprised to see how relaxed you are already. If there is any part of your body that's not yet relaxed, it soon will be. And if there's any part of your body that's not feeling as comfortable as it might, concentrate on that part of the body for the next few seconds. Just think of it and send looseness and relaxation into that area. Consciously be aware of any part of your body that's not as comfortable as it might be.

And, now, I want you to picture yourself at the top of a flight of ten stairs going down. Let's walk down these steps together and, with every step down you take, you're going to relax just a little bit more.

And, now, you can take the first step down. You've taken one step down and you have nine to go. With every step down, you relax just a little bit more. Any noise you hear will serve to relax you just a little bit more.

And now, take another step down. With every step down, you relax just a little bit more. Now you have taken two steps down and you have eight steps to go.... Take another step down, relaxing just a little bit more with every step you go down. Feel that relaxation in your body. You may be surprised at how relaxed you feel already. Now, take another step down. That's four steps down and you have six to go. This is a time for relaxa¬tion. It's not necessary for you to go to sleep but, if you want to, that's fine. If it happens, that's fine; or, if your mind drifts away, that's fine. Nothing that you do is wrong.

Take one more step down. Now you're halfway down the stairs. You have five more steps to go. Now, take another step down. See yourself on the sixth step down. See how comfortable you feel, how secure you feel and how trusting you feel. And, now, another step down.... You've taken seven steps down and you have three to go. Take another step down.... You've taken eight steps and you have two more to go. And, now, one more step.... You've taken nine steps down and you have one to go.... Now, take that last step down and you're all the way down to the bottom of the stairs. You may be surprised at how relaxed you are.

And now, I'd like you to picture yourself on a lovely, warm beach. Way out in front of you is a calm, very blue ocean: very calm and very blue. See if you can smell what the ocean smells like.

The sun is gently warming your skin, while, at the same time, you also feel a cool breeze. You feel bathed in love and fully alive. You hear the ocean lapping on the shore. Listen to what it sounds like.... Underneath your feet is the warm sand, just the right temperature, the way you like it best. Behind you is an enormous and beautiful beach....

And now, while you're standing there, imagine yourself as a little girl at a time when you were very happy, very content and very secure. Now, feel that happiness, feel that security, and soak up that carefree feeling, and know that that's you.... Remember, you can bring back this feeling of happiness and contentment any time you want to. It's your feeling. It's your memory. The only one in the world who has that memory is you.

And, now, picture yourself standing on the beach once again, as an adult. Look down and see a large, brightly coloured beach towel waiting for you on the sand by your feet. Picture yourself lying down on the towel on your back and feel how secure the ground is under you, holding your calves and your backside and your shoulders and your head. You are totally safe, secure and protected.

And now, I'd like you to imagine yourself surrounded by a lovely golden light. It covers every inch of your body. This lovely golden light is the healing power of the universe, the healing power of your own body and that golden light can go anyplace you tell it to.

While you bask in this beautiful golden light, I want to you to silently repeat aloud each line you are about to read back to yourself:

I love you dear body of mine.
You are beautiful and perfect exactly as you are: right here, right now.
You were made in the image of the Great Goddess, strong, curvy, solid, and gorgeous.
I am sorry I am so hard on you.
I am sorry I pick at you, criticize you, and put you down.
I'm going to start being kinder and gentler towards you.
You are not my enemy; you are a precious friend.

As each day passes, I come to appreciate you more and more.

Appreciate you for all of the amazing things you can do and experience.
You are truly remarkable.
Bless you, dear body of mine.

And now, I'm going to be quiet for a minute or two and, while I'm being quiet, I'd like you to really let those words sink in, deep into your unconscious. I'm going to be quiet starting now....

And now, with that powerful, vigorous, vital golden light still within you that combines all of the power of the universe and of your body, I'd like you to visualize yourself standing up on the beach. You feel rejuvenated and refreshed and nourished from the inside out.

Now, picture yourself at the bottom of the same flight of stairs you came down earlier and, together, we'11 walk up those stairs. When you reach the top of the stairs, you will be back at the place where you started, feeling completely alert while also comfortably relaxed. Now, let's take the first step up. And now the second step. And the third...and the fourth...and the fifth. You're halfway up the stairs now. Let's get to the top together by climbing the sixth step; and now the seventh, the eighth, now the ninth and, finally, the tenth.

We made it!

Take a deep breath and exhale.

Open your eyes whenever you feel ready[6]

---

6   Adapted from *Script for Guided Imagery* by Harold H. Benjamin. Refer:
    < http://www.twc-wla.org/images/Guidelmg_files/Guidelmg.htm>.

7

changing our minds

Now, we've come to what I like to call the "meat" of this entire book. Or, perhaps, I should call it the "nuts" or the "beans" for those of us who are vegetarians.

If there is one thing I've learned, both as a therapist and as a "mere" woman fumbling her way as best she can through life in the 21st century, it's that no one teaches us how to THINK properly. It absolutely amazes me, really. Take all our advancements in knowledge. Consider that we all, in this technologically savvy time in which we live, have easy access to this fund of knowledge. And yet, with a possible few rare exceptions, we are still most of us suffering from what I like to call "impoverishment of mind". We may have all the money in the world, all the success we could ever dream of and even be perfectly healthy yet still feel absolutely miserable with ourselves and our lives.

For confirmation of this, you only have to look to Hollywood. We could each of us, with very little effort, make a long list of celebrities who, to all appearances, have it all, everything required for personal happiness – fame, the adulation of an adoring public, money and all its trappings, the freedom to go where you want and do as you please, the license to indulge yourself shamelessly. But this life of pomp and privilege is, so frequently, all appearances, as deceiving as a Hollywood movie set. Look a little deeper and you'll soon see that many, even most, of these celebrities lead lives of quiet desperation – suffer from eating disorders, depression, and various addictions that frequently and repeatedly land them in rehab centers, cause them to squander their fortunes and ruin their careers. How common is the Hollywood story of the faded star!

The ruined celebrity phenomenon is, I believe, symptomatic of something that runs very deep in our society. This something is so prevalent, so rampant in our society that it amounts to what I like to refer to as the "delusion of the masses". It is the belief, the erroneous belief, that being thin, rich and famous is the formula for happiness. It's the belief that success in life is to be measured by these yardsticks – the size of your bank account, the amount of envy you arouse in others, and the size of your waist which should be inversely proportional to the size of your back account. We're all aware that this is a complete falsehood, yet we continue to hope that there is truth in this false belief. It almost seems a kind of suspension of disbelieve – like in the movies! We pretend the blood is real even though we know it isn't. How do we account for this delusion? How has it taken such a hold on society at large? How is it that each one of us has, in some measure, come under its influence? Are we just stupid? Or is there something else at work here?

Of course, it would be too simplistic to reduce this phenomenon to the general stupidity of people. The truth is, you're a pretty smart cookie. I'm a pretty smart cookie. We should all know better. But what I really think is going on here boils down to one thing and one thing only: bad training. In fact, I believe that most of the bizarre behaviors we engage in that hurt us can be attributed to bad training, to upbringing, to the way we were taught and the patterns of behavior that were established for us long before we could think for ourselves – the stuff we learned along the way to becoming adults. The wrong thinking that we acquired during those early years when we were coming of age is not easily undone, admittedly, but it can be undone and the purpose of this book is to help you start the work of undoing all those wrongheaded ideas that have led to your eating disorder. Let's focus for a bit on how our thinking can influence how we feel regarding food and our bodies.

I love the saying my mother got from a therapist she knew many moons ago: "Suffering is optional." While I don't think this can be applied to every single circumstance, I do think it is of significant value when we're talking about things that we have control over, things such as our feelings. For example, while you cannot control the outcome of a job interview, you do have some choices regarding how you deal with the outcome. Let's say you didn't get the job. You could beat yourself up emotionally and take the rejection as proof that you really are a loser and not worthy to be hired for the position; or, you could feel the initial disappointment but reason that you didn't get the job because something greater is on its way for you. I expect your mood would be a whole lot brighter were you to choose the second viewpoint. Attitude really can make a difference; it can change your view of particular circumstances and things generally, including how you feel about yourself. It can literally transform the way you view yourself, your life and your world.

Now, let's dig into the material I have prepared for you. We'll start with a discussion about how women with food and body image issues tend to think and how their thinking gets them into trouble. Then, I'd like to explore with you the most common forms of distorted thinking commonly related to eating disorders and give you some practical tools you can use to change distorted thoughts and shift your thinking from negative to positive. Lastly, I'd like to show you how to manage your thinking so that you're controlling it and not the other way around so that positive thinking becomes habitual.

Here are some of the thoughts clients with food and body image issues share with me regularly:

"Other people are looking at me and judging me based on how I look."

"I am ugly and no one will ever love me."

"I am crazy because I have food issues."

"I have to look like a supermodel to be accepted."

"I have to be perfect or else I'm not worthy of love/attention/acceptance."

You can be sure that these thoughts are not making any of the women thinking them feel better about themselves. Why? Because negative thinking leads to negative feelings, it's that simple. I like to call it the "what you think is what you get" syndrome. If you *think* you're ugly, you'll *feel* ugly. But if you think you're beautiful, you'll feel beautiful.

Negative thinking can be a vicious, self-perpetuating cycle wherein negative thoughts lead to negative feelings, which prompt more negative thoughts. The good news is, positive thinking can put you on a very happy, nurturing, self-perpetuating and self-fulfilling cycle. And the coolest part is that you don't even have to believe what you're saying to yourself because your mind isn't all that smart: now, how's that for a contradiction!

It doesn't matter if what you say is true to your brain; it only matters that you say it, frequently, repeatedly. The brain simply takes the message and sends it off, regardless of whether it's fact or pure nonsense! But, all the time, new thought paths are being carved in your brain. You're acquiring the habit of thinking positively. It's actually very simple.

Another point to be made is this: what we think is often counterproductive and downright WRONG. More often than not our thoughts about ourselves are, quite simply, mistaken. I can't tell you how true this is for me so much of the time. Since I've been working on correcting my thinking – I've come to appreciate that this is a life-long journey – I've become acutely aware of how upside-down my thinking has been for so many years! I like what 12-step programs call this phenomenon: "stinking thinking".

A great example of stinking thinking comes from a client of mine who assumed, when her husband was quiet at dinner, he was annoyed with her. When I challenged her to see if her assumption had any validity by asking him if this was actually the case, his answer surprised her. He told her that, when he was quiet at dinner, he was actually doing some deep breathing to calm himself after a stressful day at work. The purpose of his deep breathing exercises he told her was so he could fully enjoy the experience of having dinner with her and connecting at the end of the workday. In fact, he found it humorous that she thought he was annoyed with her and told her he thought that was a strange thing to assume!

Now, when they're having dinner and he's being quiet and calming himself down, she has started to take some deep breaths herself and tell herself silently that this time of day is a wonderful opportunity to relax and get centered herself. Now, she looks forward to dinner with her husband in the evenings instead of getting worked up about it.

One of the basic assumptions of Cognitive behavioral Therapy (the form of self-help we're discussing when discussing thought modification) is that how you interpret a situation greatly affects how you feel. We often think we are reacting to situations based on our feelings when what's really happening is that we are reacting to our interpretations of these situations instead.

Here's an example to demonstrate the point:

You are waiting in line at the bank at a busy time of day and, when you finally get to a teller's counter, you smile at her but she doesn't return your smile and goes about helping you with your banking very matter-of-factly, in an unsmiling and businesslike way. Here are some things you might automatically interpret from this scenario:

She can smell my garlic breath from lunch and finds it disgusting and that's why she didn't smile back.

She thinks I'm fat and gross and not worthy of smiling at.

How rude! She doesn't like her job or appreciate her customers.

The likelihood is that none of the above is actually true; they are simply possible interpretations of what could be going on for the teller in question. It is just as likely, indeed more probable, that one of the following is actually true:

It's cloudy and rainy out so she doesn't feel like smiling today, as she is prone to Seasonal Affective Disorder, otherwise known as SAD.

She's spaced out because she's so busy and forgot to smile back at you because she's overwhelmed with her work.

She has made a resolution to eat healthier foods and just had a big salad for lunch and is afraid to return your smile for fear that she has something green in between her teeth.

However rational or irrational these stories may seem on paper, do you see the difference between the stories we can make up in our heads about an event versus the actual reality of the situation?

Human beings are fabulous story-makers and fabricators of untruths. This may come in handy when you're babysitting your five-year-old niece and want to guide her to a magical fairyland, but may not be quite so useful when assuming what other people are thinking and feeling based on their behaviour.

Now, I'd like to help you familiarize yourself with specific forms of stinking thinking, clinically known as "distorted thinking". I have chosen nine examples of distorted thinking that I feel are often at work for women who struggle with food and body image issues. We'll go over each one in detail and I will give you an opportunity to examine how each of these applies to your own personal situation through writing about them in the following pages.

"All-or-Nothing" Thinking

In my opinion, this is the most common form of distorted thinking amongst women who struggle with food and body image issues. This is the type of thinking where everything is either black or white and there are no shades of gray in between. With this type of thinking, there are always only two categories that things can fall into whether "beautiful" and "ugly", "brilliant" and "stupid", or any other pair of opposites you tend to favour.

This type of distorted thinking is usually tied to having extremely high and often, unattainable standards and is often associated with perfectionist thinking.

Here's an example: a client of mine thought there were only two ways to be with food, either to be starving herself or eating everything in sight. She was either on a strict diet eating way too little or she was on an all-out binge, standing at the door of the refrigerator gorging on its contents. She was so used to these two extremes that the idea of finding a middle ground didn't even occur to her.

Do you engage in "all-or-nothing" thinking?

Write some examples below that are related to food and how you see your body.

"Should" Statements

Pardon a boast but I wear the crown on this one. I am the queen of *shoulds*. I have very clear and concise rules about how things *should* be and, if things don't go as they're supposed to —as they *should* – I am afraid the sky will fall on my head. Some people would call me a control freak and they'd probably be right to do so. For example, I think I *should* exercise every day and, if I don't, I mercilessly beat myself up for being lazy and undisciplined. A clue that you are a *shoulder* is if you often have thoughts or make statements that include the following words: *should, must, ought* and *have to*.

Do you engage in "should" thinking?

Write some examples below that are related to food and how you see your body.

Mind Reading

The practice of mind reading isn't the sole territory of people who claim to have psychic powers: most of us do this on a regular basis. We are mind reading when we make the assumption that we know what another person is thinking. We are so sure we are right that we don't bother to check out whether our assumption is correct which can lead to countless arguments and faulty conclusions.

For example, you may think that everyone is judging you and thinking you are "a tart" when you wear a tighter-than-usual top. In reality, some people may think you look lovely while others may not even notice how you look.

Do you engage in mind reading?

Write some examples below that are related to food and how you see your body.

Fortune Telling

Again, you don't have to be a professional psychic to engage in this phenomenon. Almost everyone I know does some good old fortune telling now and then when they predict the very worst by catastrophizing little things that, upon closer examination, really aren't such a big deal. People who catastrophize have a predilection for believing that something is far worse than it actually is.

For example, one of my clients received some constructive criticism from her boss on a project she was working on and had convinced herself just minutes after this conversation that she would be fired and living on the streets within the week when, in fact, her boss was pleased with the job she had done but had a few helpful suggestions to make it even better.

Do you engage in fortune telling?

Write some examples below that are related to food and how you see your body...

Personalization

Simply put, personalization is the tendency to take things personally. To give a personal meaning to the actions of others that may have nothing to do with you. I think of it, when it happens, as a kind of "selective bout of narcissism".

Personalization happens at those times when we you are so caught up in yourself that you delude yourself into thinking that something that happens externally was because of you.

For example, your girlfriend doesn't call you back right away and you assume it's because she's mad at you. However, when you do finally talk to her, she laughs when you say this and says – "But why would I be mad at you? You're my best friend. I was just crazy busy with work and the kids and this is the first chance I've had to call you back."

Do you engage in personalization?

Write some examples below that are related to food and how you see your body.

Emotional Reasoning

I'm not sure if I'm right about this but I strongly suspect more women than men suffer from this form of distorted thinking.

Emotional reasoning happens when we decide that something is true based on how we feel. I think the best example of this is when you wake up and put a nice outfit on and feel good about your appearance and then you make one not-so-great food choice at lunch and, suddenly, you begin to think you are fat.

How much you weigh hasn't changed, just how you *feel* based on an extraneous event (i.e. eating something not so healthy).

Do you engage in emotional reasoning?

Write some examples below that are related to food and how you see your body.

Labeling

I like to call this the "drama queen" syndrome.

This is when you attach a label to yourself that is inaccurate, unhelpful and often emotionally loaded. In a way, it's another form of all-or-nothing thinking in that you are making a global statement about yourself by forming a generalization that simply isn't true.

For example, you may call yourself "unattractive" when, in fact, you only dislike a couple of things about your appearance.

Labeling and generalization assists you in your irrational and negative thinking.

Do you engage in labeling?

Write some examples below that are related to food and how you see your body.

Selective Attention and Magnification

This is a classic case of seeing "the cup half empty".

Selective attention means you notice and remember certain things – the negative things – more than others. By focusing on the negative, on the little flaws, you miss out on the big picture that isn't so flawed.

A perfect example of this is obsessing on the size and shape of your body. You are never satisfied because you keep picking out things about your body that aren't "perfect" and miss out on appreciating those things that are attractive and lovely about your body.

Do you engage in selective attention and magnification?

Write some examples below that are related to food and how you see your body.

Discounting the Positives

This one essentially speaks for itself. I like to call this the "Eyore syndrome".

Do you remember Eyore, the donkey from Winnie the Pooh, who is constantly sighing with hopelessness and resignation? This is "stinking thinking" at its best.

You may have just gotten a promotion at work, your kids are happy and healthy, but you sprained your ankle and all you can focus on is not being able to walk as comfortably as you did yesterday and nothing else seems to matter.

Do you engage in discounting the positives?

Write some examples below that are related to food and how you see your body.

So, where do we go from here? We've learned that we are predominantly fueled by a way of thinking that is faulty, harmful and, simply put, "bass-ackwards". How can we start to change the way we think so that we feel more in control of our thoughts and feelings? Well, thanks to cognitive behavioural therapy, there is a lot we can do in this regard.

In this section, I'm going to give you three excellent tools to help you change your thinking for the better. The first revolves around identifying ingrained distorted thinking patterns and coming up with more positive alternatives. This is the mother of all cognitive behavioural therapy techniques; its effectiveness in altering distorted thinking patterns has been proven through practice.

The second tool will help you uncover any core beliefs you have about yourself and the world around you that are creating suffering and pain in your life so that you can examine them closely, shine a flashlight on them, have a good laugh (or cry) over them and then toss them into the garbage where they belong.

This will bring us to the last tool, one you may be familiar with already – positive affirmations. I'll give you a "can't lose" formula for creating affirmations regarding food and body image that will leave you feeling strong, empowered and at peace with yourself.

So let's dig in, shall we?

I'd like you to refer to the chart on the following page, entitled "Changing My Thinking by Having a Good Argument with Myself".

This is an adaptation of a similar chart called "the daily mood log" from David Burns's *Feeling Good Handbook*. I strongly suggest you pick up a copy of this fabulous resource on cognitive behavioural therapy. In an easy-to-follow, self-help format, this book will help you delve deeper into changing your thinking patterns in order to feel better.

But for the purposes of this book, I'll share the following exercise that you can use to get you started.

To begin, review the chart on the following page.

changing my thinking
by having a good argument with myself

Date & Time				
What Just Happened				
Automatic Distorted Thoughts I Had				
What Type of Distortion Is This				
Why this is Not True; Evidence to the Contrary				
A New Take on the Distorted Thought; Replace the Negative Thought with a Positive Thought				

Now, I'd like you to think about the past week and come up with some examples then complete a chart for each instance of distorted thinking you can recall.

What Just Happened/Automatic Distorted Thought I Had

To start each instance of distorted thinking, you'll pick an event that happened and then think back and write down the automatic thought you had when it happened. Then you'll need to review the types of distorted thinking outlined earlier to find the particular type of distortion that applies to your example and write it in the chart.

For example,

I was driving and waved to my friend who was crossing the street and she didn't wave back. My automatic thought was, "She's angry with me."

What Type of Distortion is This

Now, list the distorted thought or thoughts you had during this event. Here's a quick list of the types for your reference but don't hesitate to refer back to their descriptions if you need further reminding:

"All-or-Nothing" Thinking, "Should" Statements, Mind Reading, Fortune Telling, Personalization, Emotional Reasoning, Labeling, Selective Attention and Magnification and Discounting the Positives.

In the above example, the woman used: mind reading by assuming she knew what her friend was thinking as well as personalization when she assumed that the reason her friend didn't wave back had something to do with her.

Why this is Not True; Evidence to the Contrary

In this section, I'd like you to go ahead and have a good argument with yourself and list reasons proving why your automatic thought is faulty.

In the example given, this woman could write:

Just because she didn't wave back doesn't mean she's angry with me. Maybe she just didn't see me. We had a great time together on the weekend and she told me how valuable I am to her, so there is no reason for her to be angry with me.

A New Take on the Distorted Thought

Now, I want you to take your distorted thought and turn it around, turn the negative thought you had into a positive thought that you could replace it with in future.

Finally, in the example given, this woman could write the following affirmation:

Just because someone doesn't respond to me the way I would like them to does not mean they are upset with me. I am a wonderful friend with so much to offer and my friends respect and appreciate me and treat me well.

When we start to dissect our thinking and look at what's beneath the surface, if we dig deep enough, we'll eventually come to what are called our core beliefs. These are the generalized, global beliefs you hold about yourself, your future, or the world around you. Negative core beliefs I often hear from clients include: "I'm unlovable"; "I'm not good enough"; and "no one can be trusted". We develop these beliefs in childhood based on our experiences and what we learned from our families-of-origin growing up. These negative core beliefs have a way of sticking around; they persist and can cause countless problems for us as adults. For example, if from our mothers we learned that we are worthy only if we look a certain way, we'll keep working from that belief as adults.

The other interesting thing about core beliefs is that they are unconditional. Through them, your perception is filtered so that they affect how you see yourself, as well as others, in specific situations. The good news is that getting to the root culprit of your negative thinking (i.e. your negative core beliefs) and changing them for the better will produce long-lasting positive changes in your thinking and in your life. Once we understand what our negative core beliefs are and where they come from, we can then find ways to disregard them when they pop up into our consciousness and choose new, more life-affirming thoughts instead.

Now, I'd like to give you a helpful tool to get at your core beliefs. Pardon the psychobabble but, in therapeutic jargon, this tool is referred to the "downward arrow technique" and here is how it works.

When you have an automatic thought, apply the following formula of questions to the thought:

What's so bad about that?

What does that say about me?

Keep asking the questions until you find yourself repeating the same answer over and over again. This answer is probably a core belief for you.

Here's an example:

Julie just got an upsetting phone call from her mother who blamed her for forgetting her sister's birthday last week (Julie is 42 by the way). As soon as she gets off the phone, she eats an entire bag of pretzels. She automatically thinks, "I pigged out and now I'm stuffed and feel gross." She asks herself:

What's so bad about that?

↓

"If anyone else sees the empty pretzel bag in the garbage, they'll think I'm a pig."

↓

What's so bad about that?

↓

"If they think I can't control what and how much I eat, they will reject me."

↓

What's so bad about that?

↓

"I'll have no one to love me."

↓

What does this say about me?

↓

"I'm unlovable."

Ta da! There you have it. Julie has found her core belief. She is "unlovable".

I'd like you to try this out for yourself now. Pick one event and its corresponding automatic thought that you had written on your chart from the previous exercise. To help you along, use the downward arrow technique as used by Julie in the above example. Take each thought to the next level by repeatedly asking yourself the question "*What's so bad about that?*" and then "*What does this say about me?*" until you have come to a core belief. Write down that core belief. Keep it handy. You'll need it for the next exercise.

One of the most powerful techniques for changing our minds is creating and saying positive affirmations to ourselves repeatedly, day in and day out. I'm guessing that you've heard about positive affirmations and have experience in actually using them so you probably have an idea of what I'm talking about here.

But how I'd like to use affirmations right now is to tie them specifically to the goal of finding peace with food and your body. I use this technique almost daily in my therapy practice and have seen incredible results with those clients who use the affirmations regularly and consistently. I have seen so many women begin to see food and their bodies in an entirely different way and to start to feel good about how they eat, what they eat and how they look as a result.

There are a couple of general guidelines to creating affirmations that will produce the best results. The first is that they have to be in the present tense, not the past or future. So make them in the here and now for maximum effectiveness.

For example, this thought:

Someday I will see my body as a temple; a sacred home for my spirit and my mind.

is a lot more compelling when expressed in the present tense:

My body is a temple, a sacred home for my spirit and my mind.

The other thing to remember when creating a powerful, life-changing affirmation is to use only strong, positive words and to leave out negative, self-defeating words.

For example, this thought:

I love my eyes even though they are too close together.

is not nearly as powerful as:

I love my eyes. They are a beautiful, deep brown colour, rich and alive.

Also, keep your affirmation fairly short so that you can easily memorize it. It can be anywhere from one to five sentences. The whole thing should be able to fit onto one side of an index card when written out in full.

Here's another tip for creating affirmations: when you read them or say them out loud, they should sound "cheesy" or too-good-to-be-true or even downright ridiculous to you. They should be things that you normally wouldn't say to yourself.

The reason for this is because you are telling your brain new things that it may not even believe yet, but that doesn't matter. You are training your mind to think in new and different ways. Remember, you don't have to believe any of the things you tell yourself to gain the wonderful outcomes, which positive affirmations can bring.

For the following exercise, try writing these first in the space provided and edit them until you've got exactly what you want. Then, print each affirmation out neatly on an index card. Index cards are handy because you can easily tuck them into a wallet or daybook or even a novel and carry them around with you for easy access.

Step 1

Pick one of the core beliefs you identified in the last exercise and create a positive, life-changing and transformational affirmation to replace it.

For example, if one of your core beliefs is "I cannot survive being criticized", you could write something like:

I am a strong, incredibly bright and articulate woman with important things to say.

Anyone who has ever had anything important to contribute to society has been criticized and survived.

I invite all criticism of my ideas – bring it on! I'm ready for it!
I have wonderful counterarguments to each and every criticism that comes my way and use them when needed.

These rebuttals on my part only serve to strengthen my convictions and credibility.

Step 2

Create an affirmation for how you want to relate to food.

Here is an example of a powerful, life-changing affirmation for how a person could learn to view food:

Food is a sacred source of fuel to power my body.

Food is my friend and an ally in my healing.

Food gives me the energy I need to live my life to the fullest.

Food enables me to enjoy all of the fabulous experiences that life has to offer.

By choosing and eating healthy, life-giving food, I nourish my body, my mind and my spirit.

Step 3

Create an affirmation for how you want to see your body.

Here is an example of one I came up with:

My body is a temple, a sacred home for my spirit and my mind.

My body is perfect exactly as is, a creation of the Divine Spirit.

My body is a dear friend that allows me to experience so many things: seeing, tasting, smelling, touching and hearing.

I am so lucky to be given the gift that is my body; with each passing day, I appreciate and love my body more and more.

8

I love this body

This chapter is divided into two parts. In part one, we will explore how we, as women, have become susceptible to society's beauty standards and ideals. We'll explore the history of the development of the concept of feminine beauty in 20th century North American society and we'll look at our own personal and individual histories to see how it is that we have come under the influence of society's expectations when it comes to beauty and the female body.

In part two, we will gather some useful tools to become freer of outside pressures to look a certain way. These will include journaling exercises, writings and examples of women who courageously defy our culture's standards of beauty and success. We'll also discuss some practical tips for learning to love the body you have.

I would like to introduce this topic by taking a look at how we, as women, have been affected by our culture's beauty standards. I'll start us off by talking about myself.

I learned from a very early age that the way I looked was not considered desirable.

I had:

- Dark hair which should have been blond

- Dark brown eyes which should have been ice-blue

- Curly hair which should have been straight

- A naturally curvy and rounded body which should have been straight up and down and bony-thin

- Small shoulders when I should have had wide bony ones from which a dress or blouse could be elegantly draped

I was:

- Short and compact when I should have been tall and lanky

- Near-sighted and needed glasses because my eyes were too dry for contact lenses when I should have had perfect vision or been able to wear contacts to hide my poor eyesight

- Long in the torso and short in the legs when I should have been the other way around

Now, in the space below, I'd like you to write about how you did or did not meet the beauty ideals of the era in which you grew up.

Body image issues are a fairly recent phenomenon. Although girls have always been self-conscious about their looks, identity was not always wrapped up in the way the body looked. But the female body has always been a spectacle. It has always been moulded to fit society's expectations and to be judged. In the 19th century and beginning of the 20th, female bodies were shaped with clothing and undergarments used to hide the body's perceived flaws. If a woman did not have a naturally small waist, she used a corset to give her a small waist. Although this may have been physically discomforting, wearing a corset did not seem to do the same psychological damage that has been achieved through a historically later development – the internalization of beauty.

The internalization of beauty began in the 1920s. This was when dieting and home scales became common in North American. Before that, county fairs and drugstores were the only places where women could weigh themselves. The flapper look had become popular, emphasizing small breasts, a thin waist and narrow hips. Women saw the flapper style as a freedom because they didn't wear corsets under the short, loose flapper dresses. This is when dieting and the internalization of beauty became popular — the idea that the body can be shaped through self-control. Denying oneself food became the means to achieving the desired look.

As the industrial age began, clothing started to be mass-produced and standard clothing sizes were created. Suddenly girls had a new way to compare themselves to friends. Clothing size was no longer just how much fabric was needed; it was a number, a gauge for beauty and success. Thanks to the new sizing system, there was now a way to measure a woman and to label her based on how she "sized up". Concepts like Plus Size and Petite came into being and many women learned, to their dismay, that their bodies were not the norm. Weigh scales, the sizing system, the concept of dieting and fashion trends were little more than tools for the indoctrination of women. Women were not expected to question but only accept the beauty standard put before them.

From the 1920s right up until today, thin has been in. Companies make billions of dollars convincing women that their bodies could, and should, look better. Marketing and fashion now influences, not to say dictates, what women find beautiful. In the 1950s, the mass production of bras began and large, lifted, pointy breasts became all the rage. Exercises to increase bust size were widely published in teen magazines. "We must, we must, we must increase our bust." was the mantra for a generation of girls.

The 1950's heralded the advent of fashionable eyewear for girls and women. There was a huge boom in the design and marketing of "fashionable frames". Not only that, but contact lenses grew tremendously in popularity among teenage girls.

In the 1960s and 70s fashion models gained popularity. The word "model" itself means "the ultimate example and perfection to which all must aspire". Twiggy was the quintessential model of the time and the first to have the "waif" look.[1]

Unfortunately, not much has changed since Twiggy came on the scene. Still today, instead of celebrating womanly curves, fashion models continue to look more like adolescent girls. Since more than 97% of us are not naturally stick-thin, we end up dieting and starving ourselves to have "the look" that is still in vogue more than 30 years after Twiggy arrived.

Well, maybe things have changed a bit. It's no longer enough to simply starve ourselves – we must also be an athlete of sorts. The new look requires us to be thin yet absolutely toned. Oh, and we're also supposed to have large yet surprisingly perky breasts. Since this look is physically impossible for the majority of us, millions of women undergo plastic surgery to maintain the current beauty ideal.

Teresa Riordan, author of *Inventing Beauty: a History of the Innovations That Have Made us Beautiful*, puts it this way:

> *Exercise is seen as a virtuous pursuit. To be healthy, all people need to do is walk briskly several times a week and do a little stretching. Yet we tend to think of someone who spends two hours a day body sculpting at the gym as 'virtuous'. In fact, she is not any less vain than someone who achieves the same effect with liposuction.[2]*

1   Brumberg, Joan Jacobs. *The Body Project: An Intimate History of American Girls.* (New York: Random House, 1997).
2   Riordan, Teresa. *Inventing Beauty: A History of the Innovations that Have Made us Beautiful.* (New York: Broadway Books, 2004) 278.

And this body image obsession is not only relegated to our hips, butts, thighs and breasts. The perfect body isn't perfect if it doesn't also include those glaringly white, perfectly straight "Chicklet" teeth. Ms. Riordan calls those women who have their teeth whitened and veneered the "dentally improved" and points out that they somehow manage to escape the judgement and criticism of those who have breast implants.[3]

Riordan also points out in her book that, with the advent of high-speed technology, beauty trends are transmitted at lightning speed, a phenomenon she calls, "The Law of Accelerating Beauty". She states that, along with this phenomenon, we also have the "Principle of Age Deceleration" – i.e. forty is the new twenty.

Lastly, Riordan acknowledges that many of us worry that the current obsession with plastic surgery, this season's spectator sport on television, has turned beauty into a kind of "physiological sameness". She agrees while observing, "This trend is not unique to plastic surgery; nor is it a new phenomenon. Virtually every beauty invention that has taken flight – from corsets to cosmetics – has tended to mold Woman into a collective, ideal form. It is just that the technology has gotten a lot more effective."[4]

Paul Campos, author of *The Obesity Myth: Why America's Obsession with Weight is Hazardous to your Health*, calls this the "bimbo culture" which advertises itself as a celebration of youth, beauty and sexiness. He argues, however, that bimbo culture really has very little to do with any of those things.

---

3   Ibid, 277-8.
4   Ibid, 277.

Instead, he states that

> *our current obsession with maintaining an absurdly thin body has more to do with darker strains of that part of American culture that has always distrusted desire in general, and has now come to fear food in particular, as a harbinger of sloth, gluttony, lust and every other deadly consequence of uncontrolled indulgence in life's pleasures.*[5]

He sums it up this way:

> *Our hyper thin celebrities, whether they are entertainers or politicians – a distinction that has become increasingly meaningless – present us with images of virtuous denial: I do not eat, therefore I am (famous). Someone like Madonna, who is said to work out for several hours every day and who, for a time, entered every bite of food that went into her mouth into a computer program, could be considered a sort of secular saint of this culture: a kind of unholy anorexic, denying herself food so that we might live out our fantasies of unlimited indulgence through her.*

> *Madonna, and those like her who make up People magazine's A-list, are not so much singers or actors or journalists or politicians as they are hunger artists. In the end, the bimbo culture is essentially a culture of anorexia nervosa.*[6]

---

5   Campos, Paul. *The Obesity Myth: Why America's Obsession with Weight is Hazardous to your Health.* (New York: Gotham Books, 2004), 97-98.
6   Ibid, 97-98.

A very powerful tool to develop a more positive body image is to focus on self-supporting, rather than self-criticizing messages about your body.

Under each of the headings on the following pages, I'd like you to make a list, a list as complete as possible of all the things that belong under that heading.

What I Like About My Appearance

What Others Like About My Appearance

My Attractive Behaviours

(i.e. What is attractive about me apart from my physical appearance.)

That done, I'd like you to pick one item from your attractive behaviours list and write down a few ideas about how you could focus on enhancing and improving that aspect of your personality.

The general idea here is to tune into how you behave rather than how you look.

Next, I want you to write down one change you could make in your appearance, besides losing weight, which will enhance how you feel about yourself. For example, if you're waiting to buy clothes until you're thin, you could choose to buy something you really like now that fits you exactly as you are.

Now, I'd like to share with you my

Top 10 Tips for Loving Your Body:

1. Focus on what magnificent things your body allows you to DO rather than how it LOOKS.

2. Keep an index card in your wallet or day-timer with a list of 10 positive things about yourself excluding physical attributes. Read it over when you get "fat head".

3. Wear clothes you like that feel comfortable, especially materials that feel luxurious against your skin.

4. Throw out your thin clothes! Only keep clothes that fit you really nicely now and get rid of "the ones I'll wear when I'm a _____ size again."

5. Do the activities you love to do regardless of your shape and size – don't stop doing what you love because of what you look like on the outside!

6. Hang out with others who aren't obsessed with their size and shape and what they eat but who focus more on enjoying this fabulous gift we call life.

7. Remind yourself that you are beautiful exactly as you are because you are a child of the Creator/God/The Universe/_____(fill in the blank).

8. Move your body in ways that leave you feeling strong, exhilarated, flexible and centered – and do it regularly.

9. Learn to tune into your body: Eat when you are hungry. Rest when you are tired. Get out and move when your body needs it.

10. Stop reading fashion magazines and following movie stars, thinking they've got perfect lives. They don't. Many of them have full-blown eating disorders and the rest have something else making life no more perfect for them than it is for us regular Janes. Find alternative publications that celebrate and honour women for all aspects of their being.

Write a list of ten positive things about yourself, excluding physical attributes.

Copy this page out onto an index card and keep it in your wallet or day-timer or somewhere else where you will notice it daily. Tape it to your bathroom mirror, if you like.

Write about what clothes you like that feel comfortable, especially materials that feel luxurious against your skin.

Start wearing these clothes regularly and notice how you feel in them.

Write your feelings down.

Make a list of the clothes you own that make you feel bad about your body when you look at them or wear them.

Give them to your favourite charity and, for each item you give away, replace it with a piece of clothing like those you wrote about on the preceding page.

Write a list of all of the physical activities you enjoy doing but avoid because of how you look.

Do one of them.

Write a list of all the people you know who aren't obsessed with their size and shape and what they eat but who focus more on enjoying this fabulous gift we call life.

Try hanging out with one of these people and notice how it feels.

Write a list of all the ways you like to move your body that leave you feeling strong, exhilarated, flexible and centered.

Now do it.

Write a list of all the ways you buy into "bimbo culture" and become a victim of the media.

Come up with some strategies to lessen the effects of how the media defines you.

What are some empowering/alternative forms of entertainment you could try instead?

Make a list of movies, books, magazines, websites, etc., that will help to counter the negative influences of "bimbo culture".

Avoid some of the "bimbo culture" culprits this week and enjoy one of your alternatives from your list instead.

To inspire you, I'd like to share with you one of my favourite poems by Maya Angelou. It's called, *Phenomenal Woman*.

Phenomenal Woman

Pretty women wonder where my secret lies.
I'm not cute or built to suit a fashion model's size
but when I start to tell them,
they think I'm telling lies.
I say,
It's in the reach of my arms,
The span of my hips,
The stride of my step,
The curl of my lips.
I'm a woman
Phenomenally.
Phenomenal woman,
that's me.

I walk into a room
Just as cool as you please,
and to a man,
the fellows stand or
Fall down on their knees.
Then they swarm around me,
a hive of honeybees.
I say,
It's the fire in my eyes,
and the flash of my teeth,
the swing in my waist,
and the joy in my feet.
I'm a woman
Phenomenally.
Phenomenal woman,
that's me.

Men themselves have wondered
what they see in me.
They try so much
but they can't touch
my inner mystery.
When I try to show them
they say they still can't see.
I say,
It's in the arch of my back,
The sun of my smile,
The ride of my breasts,
The grace of my style.
I'm a woman
Phenomenally.
Phenomenal woman,
that's me.

Now you understand
just why my head's not bowed.
I don't shout or jump about
or have to talk real loud.
When you see me passing
it ought to make you proud.
I say,
It's in the click of my heels,
The bend of my hair,
the palm of my hand,
The need of my care,
'Cause I'm a woman
Phenomenally.
Phenomenal woman,
that's me.

We spend so much time focusing on how our bodies look and how they don't measure up to the latest beauty ideal but rarely do we give thanks for the functions our body provides with such ease and grace.

I'd like you to think about all the amazing things your physical body allows you to do. For example, my body carried me to work today by walking. The movement of my legs got me to my office today so that I could be here sharing this experience with you.

Now, I'd like you to complete the following:

List some of the things your body does for you in one day.

Write a short letter to your body thanking it for what it does for you and what it allows you to accomplish.

Make sure to make amends for being mean to it in the past if you have been.

closing

Well, dear reader, you made it through the entire book-congratulations! I sincerely hope that what I have presented within these pages has inspired and helped you along your journey to making peace with food and your body. If so, please share your thoughts with me and other readers by writing to: esther@estherkane.com

I wish you great success in your own personal journey.

Big hugs,

Esther

bibliography

Chapter 2 : Types of Eating Disorders

Bratman, Steven. *Orthorexia Nervosa: Overcoming the Obsession with Healthful Eating: Health Food Junkies.* New York: Broadway Books, 2000.

"Eating Disorders" *Diagnostic and Statistical Manual of Mental Disorders*, 4th edition, American Psychiatric Association, 2000: 583-595.

Chapter 3: Why Diets Don't Work

McNamara, Kathleen. *Improving Eating Behavior and Body Image: A Structured Group Program for Repeat Dieters and Others at Risk for an Eating Disorder.* Department of Psychology Colorado State University. Colorado: Fort Collins, 1986.

Poulton, Terry. *Fat Like Me.* Chatelaine September 1995: 87-105.

Chapter 4: Mindful Eating

Craighill, Peyton and Funk, Cary and Taylor, Paul. *Eating More; Enjoying Less.* Pew Research Center Publications <http://pewresearch.org/pubs/309/eating-more-enjoying-less>.

Kabat-Zinn. J. *Coming To Our Senses: Healing Ourselves and the World Through Mindfulness.* New York: Hyperion, 2005.

Kane, M. Dish: *Memories, Recipes and Delicious Bites.* Vancouver: Whitecap, 2005

Linehan, M. *Skills Training Manual for Treating Borderline Personality Disorder.* New York: Guilford Press, 1993.

Pollan, Michael. *In Defense of Food: An Eater's Manifesto.* New York: The Penguin Press, 2008.

Vangsness, Stephanie. *Mastering the Mindful Meal.* Brigham and Women's Hospital http://www.brighamandwomens.org/healtheweightforwomen/special_topics/intelihealth0405.aspx?subID=submenu10.

Weil, A. and Daley, R. *The Healthy Kitchen: Recipes for a Better Body, Life and Spirit.* New York: Knopf, 2002.

Chapter 5: The Food-Mood Connection

Brownmiller, S. *Femininity.* London: Paladin, 1984.

Mallinger, A. and DeWyze, J. *Too Perfect: When Being in Control Gets Out of Control.* New York: Fawcett Columbine, 1992.

Webb, D. *What's Eating You?* New Woman March 1998: 50-52.

SARK. *Succulent Wild Woman: Dancing with Your Wonderful Self!* New York: Fireside, 1997.

http://www.betterhealth.vic.gov.au/bhcv2/bhcarticles.nsf/pages/Depression_and_exercise?OpenDocument

http://www.truestarhealth.com/members/cm_archives03ML4P1A98.html

http://www.physicsforums.com/showthread.php?t=39324

Chapter 6: Meditation and Relaxation

Brahm, Ajahn. *Mindfulness, Bliss and Beyond.* Massachusetts: Wisdom Publications, 2006.

David, Marc. *The Slow Down Diet: Eating for Pleasure, Energy and Weight Loss.* Rochester: Healing Arts Press, 2005.

Vardey, Lucinda (Ed). *The Flowering of The Soul: A Book of Prayers By Women.* Canada: Alfred A. Knopf, 1999.

Wikipedia, The Free Encyclopedia *Hatha Yoga.* <http://en.wikipedia.org/w/index.php?title=Hatha_yoga&oldid=253525987>

Williamson, Marianne. *Illuminata: Thoughts, Prayers, Rites of Passage.* New York: Random House, 1994.

Chapter 7: Changing Our Minds

Burns, David D. *The Feeling Good Handbook.* New York: Plume, 1990.

Wilhelm, Sabine. *Feeling Good About The Way You Look: A Program for Overcoming Body Image Problems.* New York: The Guildford Press, 2006.

Chapter 8: Body Image

Brumberg, Joan Jacobs. *The Body Project: An Intimate History of American Girls*. New York: Random House, 1997.

Campos, Paul. *The Obesity Myth: Why America's Obsession with Weight is Hazardous to your Health*. New York: Gotham Books, 2004.

Riordan, Teresa. *Inventing Beauty: A History of the Innovations that Have Made us Beautiful*. New York: Broadway Books, 2004.